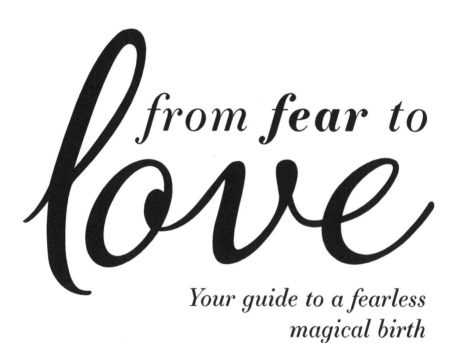

from *fear* to *love*

Your guide to a fearless magical birth

RED MILLER

Praise

'*From Fear to Love* is an amazing collection of wisdom brought to you by midwife, Red Miller. Red is a captivating storyteller, guiding you to re-evaluate the joys and challenges in life as a means to prepare for birthing with love, power, and celebration. Drawing from her experience attending births around the world, Red provides real life knowledge of pain, healing and self-discovery for preparing to experience the magic of new life. The stories are shared with a raw openness that truly honors the challenges of life while providing opportunities to help us to transform and heal to bring more love to life and birth.'

Debra Pascali-Bonaro, Director of Orgasmic Birth: The Best Kept-Secret and founder of Pain to Power Online Childbirth Class

'*From Fear to Love* is an excellent journey that every woman must imbibe as motherhood hails. It's a book from the depths of the heart of a soul who wants the best and only the very best for mothers. Thank you very much for this gem and thank you to the almighty for allowing our paths to cross.'

J Ravichandran, Consultant Obstetrician and Gynaecologist, President of the Obstetrical and Gynaecological Society of Malaysia

'I was excited when I first heard about this book – even the title made my heart soar. For years, I've been speaking about the fear that's engrained in maternity services; maternity workers are afraid, in addition to the women and families they serve. This fear leads to defensive practice and potential over-medicalisation of childbirth. *From Fear to Love* brings hope by offering solutions to help to counteract being afraid, through enhancing our ability to care, and to love.'

Sheena Byrom OBE, Midwife Consultant

'Coming from a long line of home-birthers, Red offers a great formula to turn your birth from one based in fear to one of love. As an amazing world traveller and pioneer, she brings beautiful word medicine to you. Red makes a heroic effort to help all women have a beautiful birth journey. This is a must-read book for all pregnant moms and their support people. I highly recommend it!'
Jan Tritten, Midwife, Founder and Editor-in-chief of *Midwifery Today* magazine

'At a time when birth seems dominated by fear, it is important for women and their loved ones to have a beautifully written and lively book like this to help them on their journey to becoming mothers. A journey that needs preparation, strength and awareness, as well as the understanding and awareness to get the right care providers. One of the main aims of midwifery is to support the bond of love between mother and baby, baby and parent and family. Fear spoils this love. Red has drawn from her own experience in life, as a midwife and of pregnancy, to act as guide. I love the 'mother shares' giving a sense of community, I love the focus on the experience of the baby, I love the guide to self-care and encouragement to self-love. Red's explanation of interventions is also helpful in negotiating and being involved in decisions about your care. This book will help you work through fear, contain it, and make having a baby a positive, magical experience.'
Professor Lesley Page CBE, President, The Royal College of Midwives

'Reading this book, I feel the connection Red has with her mothers and their pregnancies. She has been able to express everything the pregnant mother expects out of their pregnancy and labor. It is a book that has long been waiting to be published and I am glad it has now come into fruition. I am sure every pregnant mother reading this book will feel empowered to handle their pregnancy and labor and more importantly have a more positive experience from it all.'
Dr. Paul SL Tseng Consultant OBGYN TLC Gynaecology Practice, Medical Director Gleneagles Hospital, Assisted Reproductive Centre (GEHARPC)

'*From Fear to Love* is an exceptional debut, unique in its midwifery-led style, which contemplates aspects of pregnancy and postpartum that you won't find in any other book. This is a pregnancy bible that will tug at your heart for various reasons, be it the amazing journey of Red Miller the wonderful midwife to the power that she asks everyone to seek out during this transformative time – pregnancy, birth and new mothering.'

Priyanka Idicula, Midwife, Co-Founder and Director of Birthvillage, The Natural Birthing Center, Kerala, India

RETHINK PRESS

Contents

Introduction   1

SECTION 1   Blossoming   11

Chapter 1   Embracing Responsibility   13

Chapter 2   Pregnancy As An Opportunity For Self-discovery   22

Chapter 3   TIPS – Building Your Team   33

Chapter 4   TIPS – The Role Of Intuition   40

Chapter 5   TIPS – Partnership Health Care   45

Chapter 6   TIPS – Making Time For Self-love   54

Chapter 7   The VAGUS Model   67

Chapter 8   Working With Fear Guides   85

Chapter 9   Parenting Before Birth   92

Chapter 10   Nutrition   103

SECTION 2   Opening   113

Chapter 11   What Does Your Baby Want?   115

Chapter 12   Birth Interventions   125

Chapter 13   Stretching And Preparing To Open   136

Chapter 14   Setting The Stage   147

Chapter 15   Labor – The Bridge   156

Chapter 16   Pain And The Tools To Cope   163

Chapter 17   Everything Water   170

Chapter 18   Birth Partners   181

Chapter 19   Birth   195

Chapter 20   Surgery   203

SECTION 3 A Whole New World   **211**

Chapter 21 The Fourth Trimester   213
Chapter 22 Intuition– Responding To Your Baby's Needs   225
Chapter 23 Breastfeeding And The First Three Days   230
Chapter 24 Newborn Care   240
Chapter 25 Self-Love And Postnatal Healing   250
Chapter 26 Working Through Challenges   259

Further Resources   269
Acknowledgements   273
The Author   275

Dedicated with love to every woman who has invited me into her sacred birthing space and taught me everything I know about the process.

And to all the wonderful women and men around the world who have committed their lives to the world of birth work – I bow to you.

Introduction

"That which you seek is seeking you."

Rumi

Over the past twelve years I have learned a lot about what it takes to prepare for a healthy, positive and joyful birth; the couples I work with have been amazing teachers.

I have journeyed with thousands of women through their pregnancies and attended hundreds of births, and within that experience, like a kaleidoscope, a pattern has emerged – a pattern that has become a formula, one that shifts the experience of birth from fear to love, from the hands of a care provider, to the hands of the parents. That formula is what I want to share with you.

Belief in birth as a normal event is also ingrained in my bones. I am very blessed to come from a long line of women who believe deeply in the normality, the power of natural birth: I grew up in a community in the middle of the woods in northern Canada, where my mum was the community midwife and my grandmother gently gave birth to 14 children.

For as long as I can remember, I have always been fascinated by the magic of pregnancy. I used to study pregnant women in my community and later those out and about in my town; they were the most magical creatures I could imagine. What would it feel like to grow another person inside your body? How is that even possible? What would it feel like when they wriggle and stretch, and what would it be like to be that little person, warm and safe and constantly carried by the mother?

There are many things deemed magical in childhood that seem to fade as time passes; imagination diminishes in the face of facts, figures, and the daily norms of life. However, for me, this one magical fascination has never gone away. Being a midwife is the most incredible job I can imagine because I get to surround myself with that childhood magic. I still feel the same way: in awe of this process.

The power of love and the need to follow my heart and my gut have been other central themes in my life.

I moved away from my home to Mexico when I was 18, with a boy I had fallen in love with. I joined the circus some time in my early 20s and toured for four carnival seasons. I spent each off-season travelling around New Zealand, Guatemala and Central America, Mexico, and Europe. I always travelled alone and without any real plan. At one point, I lived in London for three years or so because I fell in love again – the trip was only meant to be for a couple weeks. However, my heart had other ideas, months turned into years, and I didn't feel the need to go anywhere else.

My move to Singapore, from where I write these words, was also for love but this time it was different. It is a mature love, one still bursting with passion but with a different feel; one that comes from age, experience, and a clear idea of what matters in life. Before Singapore, I had been living in India for five years and was on my way to establishing a second natural birth center in Bangalore. But when this love came knocking, I followed my heart's desire without looking back. Four years later we are married and expecting our first child. My heart has found its home.

Magic and love are the two main ingredients I wish for the world to keep in mind when they think of pregnancy, birth and becoming a mother.

Writing this book has been an incredibly special experience because in parallel I was going through IVF, and finally experiencing the magic of pregnancy for myself. Feeling a person wiggling and squirming inside *my* body has not been a disappointment.

I feel better, sexier, and stronger than ever now that my body is made up of four arms, four legs, two hearts – and possibly even a penis and little balls! I am a magic genie!

Each passing week, feeling those rolls, then kicks, becoming stronger and stronger, I know that my body is sustaining and nurturing a person who has decided to come and join my tribe, our family: someone who wants to walk with us into this life and teach us to remember that magic is everywhere, someone who will completely change my life and the lives of everyone I know and love.

Different cultures, different births

Since 2007, when I finished my training and got my license to practice as a Certified Professional Midwife (CPM), I have worked in homes, public health centers, birth centers and hospitals. While I have mostly practised alone, I've also worked in group practices and often with other midwives with whom I don't share a spoken language. I have stood beside hundreds of women as they gave birth, celebrated with blooming families, and mourned with others. I have been living and practicing in Asia for more than a decade, and been so blessed to attend over 700 births in diverse settings, from the foothills of the Himalayas, to rice fields in Cambodia, to a palace in Malaysia. I have 'caught' babies in more than ten countries.

In 2010, I co-founded a birth center in Kerala, south India, named Birthvillage, with a passionate local doula and birth educator, Priyanka. Birthvillage is a center, run by midwives, that offers water birth and welcomes husbands to participate fully in the process of pregnancy and birth. Last year our gentle birth rate was 97.9% and Priyanka is now a certified midwife.

Working in such diverse settings I can see how differently each culture approaches birth, and how different levels of affluence bring their own challenges. In rural Cambodia, laboring women travel to the health center on the back of a bullock cart or scooter, or they walk, or ride a bike. They come with their families, sisters, mothers, and husbands. They like to stay outside, walking around, pausing during contractions, maybe bending down and holding onto their knees, leaning against a tree or on a shoulder for support. When the baby is ready to be born, they walk in, get up on the table, and push their babies out. Most of the relatives stay outside, lighting incense and offering bananas to the spirit house in the garden. After giving birth, they want to go home so they can cook dinner for the older children and family members who have been working in the fields all day. Birth to them is normal, something that happens between lunch and dinner.

In rural India, laboring women are surrounded by their women friends. Their husbands usually aren't allowed inside because the birth rooms are communal, and birth is seen as women's work. I rarely ever heard a sound, and even in the height of labor's intensity, barely a toe would curl. When the baby emerged, mothers didn't want to hold them immediately, or sometimes even look at them. I found that so strange, but it was true for the large majority in the rural tribal areas where I worked. They first wanted to finish with the placenta, get stitches, get their dress pulled down and get off the table.

It all felt very transactional, probably because the midwives were rushing them as there were other women waiting for the beds. Perhaps their sisters and friends had told them the quieter they were, the less fuss they made, the faster they would get out of there and the better chance they would have of avoiding a scolding or a slap from the midwife. The mums were given space later, on the postnatal wards, to take their babies gingerly check all their fingers and toes, smile and coo, and kiss their curly black heads.

Women in private hospitals in major Asian cities often cry out for an epidural before active labor starts, and they have a whole stream of interventions, including forceps and Caesareans, to pull the babies out. When the mothers are handed their babies, they often have difficulty bonding, because they feel cheated into an experience they didn't want, didn't understand, and consequently feel violated by. This lack of connection is often intensified as mothers-in-law, mothers, or older aunties take over and bathe and powder the newborns. In some cases, the baby comes to mum only at feeding time, and even then the new mummy is often told she doesn't have enough milk or that she isn't handling the baby correctly.

A few days ago, in Singapore, a teen mum in the free mums' group I facilitate told me how, during the birth, the nurse who delivered her baby gave her an episiotomy. Very casually, the nurse said that because she "was a 'C' class patient" she would need to wait for over an hour until the doctor turned up to do her stitches. I have seen how large these episiotomies are, and I can imagine the extent of the blood loss from a procedure that wasn't necessary to begin with, and was then left unfinished because of her "patient class". I wondered if that was partly why her milk was delayed in coming in, but she thought it was because the nurses had started the baby on formula right away...

More and more of Singapore's affluent women are opting for home birth. I often work with women at the top of their professional fields – scientists, doctors, bankers, lawyers, leaders of large corporations – who chose to take charge the decision-making process, opting out of institutionalized birth altogether.

I recently worked with a young Singaporean woman who was having her second baby. She wanted something different from what she had experienced the first time round; she wanted to be in charge and make her own decisions.

She managed to convince her husband, her in-laws (who she was living with), and her doctor that she would have her baby in her own bedroom, in a bath of warm water.

Several months later I sat next to her through her quiet and beautiful labor. Her husband sat cross-legged on their family bed with their two-year-old son in his lap. With the last birth surge, the baby was born. As the mother lifted her daughter up out of the water, the baby's father had tears streaming down his face and looked at her in utter amazement. Her mother-in-law was leaning against the doorframe, also in tears, and they said almost in unison 'That was the most incredible thing I have ever seen', while the proud new mum in the bath was absolutely beaming.

The philosophy of birth

Too often, regardless of setting, the key ingredients of respect, kindness and compassion are missing. Medical procedures are rarely fully explained– what the benefits, the risks, and the alternatives are; and sadly, women's voices are often silenced when they question what they are told, making true, informed consent impossible. How we are treated during the crucial time of birth is not only a women's health issue, it is a human rights issue.

Every woman, and every birth, has shaped who I am as a midwife and for that I feel honored and grateful. Every experience of birth has left me amazed, inspired and humbled by how incredibly strong women are. Being a midwife helps me stay present in the moment, in the here and now. It has pushed me to trust the skills of my hands, the accuracy of my intuition, and the strength of my heart. Compassion, patience and kindness are some of the biggest skills needed for this unpredictable work. We need to be humble, to be able to be wrong, to know there is something much bigger than us at work. We need to ground and breathe and be incredibly calm under pressure. Every birth is so different that you can never predict with any certainty what is coming next.

There are many types of midwives in the world: we do not all have the same skills or the same philosophy. I call the type of midwifery I practice biodynamic midwifery. The most familiar use of the word "biodynamic" defines a farming concept developed in 1920 by Rudolf Steiner. He described it as "a holistic understanding of the agricultural process". I love his vision of working with soil, plants and animals to boost the fertility of the land naturally, creating a balanced ecosystem. This feels exactly how I want to work with women and babies.

A biodynamic relationship is not about taking; it is about giving. I learned a lot about the principles of biodynamics while studying to become a licensed and registered biodynamic craniosacral therapist (BCST). I completed my two-year diploma training with the International Institute of Craniosacral Balancing and feel incredibly grateful to my teachers, who had a profound connection to the method and the magic of the work.

These biodynamic principles are the supporting pillars of my midwifery practice.

Pillar 1: Holistic approach
Caring for a woman physically during pregnancy is not enough her emotional, mental and spiritual wellbeing is equally important. Each one of us is as much our thoughts as our physical matter. I am committed to providing the natural remedies for common discomforts that have the least impact on the sensitive ecosystem of the mother–baby body. Using positive language to increase the mother's confidence and to reduce her fear is essential in this model of practice.

Pillar 2: Relationship of trust
First we learn to trust ourselves so we can then trust those around us. Relationships are key in midwifery: the relationship and relatedness of the mother and baby, in the primary couple, of the family to the practitioner, and of the practitioner to the family. Putting an emphasis on all four of these relationships creates better outcomes.

Pillar 3: A guiding intelligence
Health is always present in the body, regardless of what else is happening. The practitioner is not the hero, or the main attraction; they are only there to help create an environment in which the body's own inner wisdom and innate intelligence can shine. We are there to give recommendations, not tell the mother what to do, and to give the mother the ownership and the responsibility in every situation.

Pillar 4: Value of touch as nutrition

Respectful touch is an essential nourishment for the body, as well as for the mind and spirit. Kind and loving touch is a thread that crosses all cultural boundaries. We use hands not machines.

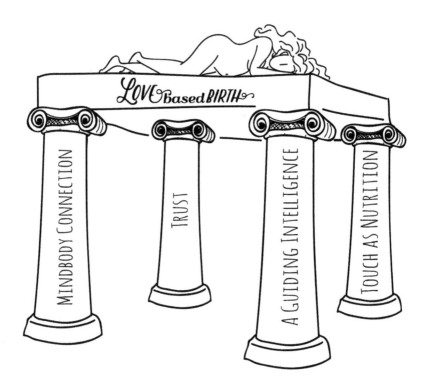

Throughout this book you will hear from women who will share with you glimpses of their experiences of becoming mothers. They are all women who I have had the pleasure of accompanying along their journey, either as their midwife for birth or as their birth preparation guide. Having their voices represented in this book is incredibly important to me because it is each of them (and so many more), who have been my teachers. Without them, this book that is now in your hands, couldn't exist.

From fear to love

Today there is a fixation in our family, friends, communities, and the media with portraying birth as a horrific drama story, one filled with pain, trauma and life-threatening circumstances in a highly medically managed hospital environment.

There is a heightened sense of "the hero" coming through, either as mother and baby conquering the odds, or as the doctor saving the day. This portrayal has consequences: it becomes a self-fulfilling prophecy as women experience more interventions that might not have even been medically necessary, creating more drama and trauma. How can birth be such a threatening process when we have the most advanced medical techniques at our disposal?

A love-filled birth is one in which fear is only an opportunity to highlight areas that the mother needs to prepare for. Mother and care provider share a commitment to get to a place of readiness, confidence, and leadership, seeing every moment of the event as something to embrace and appreciate.

Through this exploration of action and willingness to take responsibility, we begin to unlock the areas of restriction and to open more space in the body to experience greater levels of love and acceptance. This shift enables magic to happen, the body to respond innately, so we can bring our children into the world in love, celebration, and joy.

My wish for you is that with this book in your hand, you will feel like you have a biodynamic midwife at your side, cheering you on even if there is no midwife in your village, town or city. My aim is to inspire you to take good care of yourself above everything else, and to start, or continue, to build your confidence so you can have the most magical birth possible. No matter what twists and turns come up during the process of your becoming a mother, I want you to feel respected, listened to, entitled to have options and choices. I want you to feel like the most important person in the room. Whatever location you choose to give birth in, I want you and your baby to have the best experience possible. This is not only about natural birth, it is about positive birth.

I cannot guarantee you that reading this book will give you the outcome of an orgasmic water birth, but I can guarantee you that your chances of having one will be much greater, and that when you face challenges you will have the tools to face them with love and acceptance.

Lots of love and joy to you as you continue on this beautiful journey. May we all find deeper levels of kindness and compassion for ourselves each day. May we rest in knowing our ability to birth and parent is innate already within us. And may we all be confident, informed and connected parents for the next generation.

Update: While this manuscript was with the publisher I gave birth to my beautiful son Rumi Eli. Together we worked through a blissful 24 hours of labor at home; we danced, we swayed, we chanted, we sang, we aumed, we laughed, we cried; it was pure magic.

Stepping into the warm pool of water when baby was getting close was a dream come true. We were blessed with many twists and turns along the way and ultimately met our boy via Caesarean.

The experience was a gift that embodied the knowledge that the outcome, i.e. route of birth, isn't ultimately the point; I felt loved, heard, and respected throughout the entire process and that is what made my birth truly fearless and magical.

SECTION 1

Blossoming

CHAPTER 1

Embracing Responsibility

"For far too many, pregnancy and birth is still something that happens to them rather than something they set out consciously and joyfully to do themselves."
Sheila Kitzinger, author *Rediscovering Birth*

Today, the large majority of women are terrified of giving birth. Just this week a healthy young woman called me to say she was so afraid of natural birth that she was considering scheduling a Caesarean. She sounded desperate as if I were a rescue hotline – she said she hoped I could convince her otherwise as she knew there were benefits for her baby to be born from her vagina. We set up an appointment but she messaged me the next day: "Please cancel. I am too scared. There is no point in us meeting."

Fear now rules the decision-making process at one of the most critical, most magical times of our lives. I see two major problems with that:

1. Parents are giving away their power and rights too easily to a very medicalized system of doctors, midwives, nurses, and hospitals..

2. The use of largely unnecessary interventions like Caesareans, labor induction, epidurals, vacuum delivery, antibiotics and episiotomies is skyrocketing.

As a midwife, I am happy these interventions exist because they give options in emergency situations and can be life-saving. The problem is their overuse and popularity, neither of which is improving outcomes for mums and babies. In fact, they are doing the opposite, creating more complications, more Caesareans, and more lifelong health problems for our children. Health researchers are currently exploring the possibility that babies born by Caesarean are at higher risk of auto-immune conditions such as allergies, asthma, eczema, and type 1 diabetes.[1, 2] Too many mums are going home from the hospital feeling violated and confused. Postnatal depression rates today are estimated to be as high as three out of every ten new mothers.

The solution to what is becoming a global health crisis is simple:

1. Midwives and other health care professionals need to care for women in ways that build their confidence, and encourage them to connect to their power.

2. Women and couples need to make it a priority to seek out care providers who will do exactly that, and not settle for ones who continually increase their fear and confusion. We need to get better at sticking up for ourselves and our babies, saying no, and speaking our truth.

Birth is a formative experience that has the power to shape our identity as women. It is also the first opportunity for our babies to experience trust. When we give away the decision-making process, we give away our basic right, our voice and our power; that leaves us

....

[1] Caesarean section is associated with an increased risk of childhood-onset type 1 diabetes mellitus: a meta-analysis of observational studies.
Cardwell CR, Stene LC, Joner G, Cinek O, Svensson J, Goldacre MJ, Parslow RC, Pozzilli P, Brigis G, Stoyanov D, Urbonaite B, Sipetić S, Schober E, Ionescu-Tirgoviste C, Devoti G, de Beaufort CE, Buschard K, Patterson CC
Diabetologia. 2008 May; 51(5):726-35.
[PubMed]
[2] Caesarean delivery and risk of atopy and allergic disease: meta-analyses.
Bager P, Wohlfahrt J, Westergaard T
Clin Exp Allergy. 2008 Apr; 38(4):634-42.
[PubMed]

feeling victimized and incompetent, and causes our babies to suffer unnecessarily. Being connected to our maternal intuition and exercising our power is more important than ever. Saying no and exploring other options when we intuitively feel something isn't right are crucial for a positive birth outcome.

What if we started treating ourselves like the magical genies we are? Remember our ancestors and other cultures across the planet, the hundreds of millions of women who have gone before us and birthed their babies with few resources and a lot of determination? Think back to what your mum, your aunties and your grandmothers told you about their births. What was their experience? If you have never had these conversations, I encourage you to seek out the older women in your family and start asking questions. It will give you an understanding of what might subconsciously be a part of your belief around birth.

We are today in the most advantageous time for giving birth; there is no excuse for us to not be standing front and center, and leading the process. Not only do we have the intuition passed on by our foremothers, we also have the support of modern technology and evidence-based care. We can combine these two great forces to help us achieve positive, joyful and healthy birth experiences.

I asked some women I've worked with over the last year what birth taught them. They each had different types of births; many were at home, some in the hospital, and some had intervention, but most did not. This is what they had to say.

> "Birth taught me how powerful I am, and what a gift I have from God...there couldn't be a more beautiful moment."

> "Women are capable and strong, and able to handle intense pain."

> "I now know the female body is a wonderful machine that we should respect and promote."

> "To live each day without fear."

"I finally learned to let go."

"Birth taught me so many things that I could write a book! One of the greatest learnings was that we are really not alone. When a woman births, she has the strength, grace, love, support and wisdom of billions of women before her; her birth allows her to enter the infinite, unseen stream of countless Mothers before her. Birth allowed me to add my thread to the Great Tapestry, to become part of the Whole, in a way I had not known previously."

"Riding the waves is much more enjoyable than trying to lead them."

"Birth taught/showed me how amazing it is to be a woman and how to soften more with the difficult stuff."

"Listen to your core wisdom. Relax and turn towards freedom as often as you can. Search for the deep quiet free voice inside you...its the only 'right' and it brings sweet peace."

"My body is strong and capable! I have a new appreciation for what I can do, more confidence in myself and my ability to nurture life, and do something hard."

"It taught me to trust in my body. That even when I think I cannot do it myself, my body intrinsically knows what to do. Even when birthing a breech baby!"

"I am stronger and braver than I ever imagined, I am a life giver!"

"Birth taught me how strong women really are, and how powerful our minds and bodies are."

"The human body is incredible. We have been made with such divine power from God. We need to appreciate just what a miracle life is! I'm humbled. Truly."

"Birth is a miracle and one of the most precious moments in life."

"I feel like my body is flipping amazing! Seriously, I grew another human without any conscious effort from me. Then I birthed him beautifully. I'm so proud of myself, my partner, my son, and my family who were with me. I have always been a life-long feminist, but birth just gave me a whole new understanding at a very visceral level of how incredible we are as women!"

"I have so much confidence now knowing that if I can do that, I can do anything. And that sometimes birthing CAN go as planned when you are surrounded by people who support it."

"Birth is the ultimate teacher. It's the beginning of motherhood, it's the lesson that you are capable of greatness and have a strength in you that you never even knew existed, but that the cellular memory in your body knew all along that you were capable of such a feat – your body shares this wisdom with you at birth. It's an experience that becomes firmly etched in your memory forever. It creates a connection with all of womankind as well. I love that about birth – the feeling of connection with all the women who have gone before you and done this."

"Birth taught me to be wide open like the sky."

Birth can be enjoyable

I was with a mum yesterday who had come for a biodynamic craniosacral session for herself and her baby two weeks after the birth. This was her third baby, and the second birth we had been through together. She told me with tears in her eyes, "Red, sometimes I get the blues that birth is over. I feel sad I can't get those moments back, when that new life is on your chest and looking up at you, the rush of emotions and hormones. It is the most magical experience in life, and I feel so sad I will never experience that again."

As I prepare for my own birth, I feel incredibly blessed to hear experiences like this all the time.

I have learned a lot about what it takes to prepare for a healthy, natural, and joyful birth; the couples I work with have been amazing teachers.

In this first section of the book, I will share with you what they have taught me in a simple model called TIPS:

Team Building	How to build an aligned support team
Intuition	How to hear, trust and follow our intuition
Partnership Health Care	How to partner with our care providers and play a leading role
Self-love	How to slow down and care for ourselves

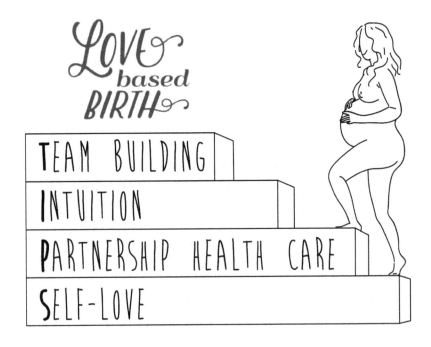

Women who follow the TIPS process use words like these to describe their experience of birth:

Magical
Empowering
Love
Partnership
Supernatural
Astral
A high
Powerful

Let's begin. First, we need to start creating intentions and building a vision for your birth. The following questions will help:

- What are the top three words that describe my ideal birth experience?

- What are the top three things I imagine my baby wants to experience from this birth?

- Where do I imagine giving birth? In what type of setting?

- Who do I see there with me?

- What are the top three most important things that I want to happen?

- What role do I imagine my partner having?

- How do I want to feel before, during and after the birth? For example:

Joyful	Respected
Connected	Open
Loved	Happy
Passionate	Prepared
Flexible	Confident
Ecstatic	Triumphant
Strong	Relaxed
Supported	Powerful

The blossoming time of pregnancy allows us gradually to start setting intentions for the birth. Once we have those in place, we can begin the work of softening, releasing and preparing to go with the flow. Intentions need to come before releasing into the flow.

> **Note:** Keep in mind that there is no right or wrong way to 'do' pregnancy, birth or new mothering. There is only your way.

Approaching birth is often described as approaching a vast mountain range a range that you can't avoid crossing. You can't be sure beforehand whether you'll be guided along the slow and steady path, which you will have to traverse back and forth as you zigzag your way up, or the opposite path, taking you up the sheer face – the most intense route but a big time saver. Preparing for any possible route is the goal, so that you feel proud and strong, regardless of the outcome.

Sticking with our analogy, you might choose to ride a horse all the way up, to have a horse available in case you need it, or not have a horse at all but have a few key people in place who you trust to carry your bags. They might carry them throughout the trip or they might be ready to take them only when you ask for their support. You might also have people available to set up your rest camps and do all the cooking, so the only thing you need to think about is putting one foot in front of the other.

Do

- Start setting your vision for how you want to feel during your birth.
- Ask your mum, your aunties and your grandmothers about their births.

- Ask yourself the following questions:

  - What are the top three words that describe my ideal birth experience?

  - What are the top three things I imagine my baby wants to experience from this birth?

  - Where do I imagine giving birth? In what type of setting?

  - Who do I see there with me?

  - What are the top three most important things that I want to ensure happens?

  - What role do I imagine my partner having?

  - How do I want to feel before, during and after the birth?

CHAPTER 2

....

Pregnancy As An Opportunity For Self-discovery

"Don't let your birth experience be stolen because you were afraid."
Dr Fred Cummings MD/OBGYN

Self-discovery and transformation are areas I have been exploring in depth since my twenties. I was blessed early in life with several major opportunities to rise like a phoenix from dark dank spaces. I am grateful and proud today to look back over my journey so far and say rise is exactly what I did.

The first opportunity came in the form of ending my love affair with cocaine, hallucinogenic drugs, alcohol and other methods of disassociation. I did it, mostly on my own with the help of my guides and angels, in my early twenties. My addiction to 'numbing out' was the same as it is for many: I had an overwhelmed nervous system that couldn't deal with the daily ups and downs because I was holding on to trauma; living my life feeling unworthy and unsafe. Sexual violation as a child; and rape and emotional abuse as a young woman, were big contributors.

The second opportunity came somewhere in my early thirties. A nervous breakdown, panic attacks and repeated loud voices from somewhere deep inside urging me to jump off my 17th floor balcony or swerve my moped into oncoming traffic nearly did me in. I was burnt out.

Burn out, sadly, is very common in the caring professions. Often women who choose to care for people have a huge capacity to give and to serve, and too often forget the importance of filling up their own cups to make that service sustainable. I was in my fifth year of living and working in a culture that was so different from my own that I was gradually losing track of who I was. I had just ended a relationship with someone I was deeply in love with but had no future with. I was completely broke and saw no way out of the pain and the loneliness, and I was desperate for ease and to feel cared for.

In both situations, I used self-love in the form of movement, yoga, affirmations, meditation, prayer, visualizations, travel, breath work, study and bodywork to explore into my own heart and soul. I was also blessed to have loving friends that I could reach out to. The practice of self-love and acceptance never stops and instead is a daily, sometimes hourly, process.

I am so grateful for the learning provided by those times in the dark because they have given me the gift of knowing the light. I know my strength, the power inside me, my ability to survive and thrive. That knowledge feels essential in my work with women. It has given me a confidence that helps me to stand in the fire with them, to look them straight in the eyes and say, "you can do this", because I know they can. We all can.

A time of transformation

The moment you see that positive line on your pregnancy test everything changes. Everything is suddenly up for question. What was I thinking? Will I be able to handle this? Will I be a good mum? Will I still be me? How will my life change? As our bodies begin to change, so does everything else. Our relationships, our priorities, our concept of self, perhaps even how we feel in the world. We are almost between worlds, right along with our growing babies – maybe seen by society as a vessel or an object, as strangers suddenly feel they have permission to comment on – we are surely either too big or too small or too energetic or too casual – or touch our bodies.

I was in my 23rd week when I started to notice that the world was beginning to see me differently. My taxi drivers wanted to chat and congratulate me, my friends wanted to carry my bags, and people stared at my boobs and my belly when I passed by. Sometimes it was as if I was in a private club when another blossoming mamma and I caught each other's eyes on the street, and we smiled and nodded, silently acknowledging each other's blossoming.

This period of transformation is not all roses and it can shake the most confident person into uncertainty. It can bring up all sorts of deep-rooted feelings of inadequacy, doubt, guilt, and blame. And there is nowhere to hide from it all because the process keeps moving forward; there is no turning back. This very nature of pregnancy provides a great opportunity to discover how to find ease in the storm as we shift from being self-focused towards nurturing and creating space for another.

"I think one of the best things that came out of the pregnancy and birth was reconnecting with my own body. It was probably one of the healthiest and most vibrant times of my life both physically and mentally. For me, I enjoyed the pregnancy and could work through my seventh month giving massages and enjoying others' company at work. I loved that I still could chop wood, take care of my horses, work at a spa, and live with enthusiasm throughout the pregnancy."
Kelly, first baby, America

While we are busy getting into our heads, there is a great deal of magic happening in the body. You are growing an entirely new human, and it is happening without you needing to do too much besides continuing to live life. What if we had the tools to live more in the magic and less in the worry? How can we begin to surrender to the process and the potential of the moment? How will we benefit, and what benefit will our baby receive? How can we daily, in small ways, build up confidence in ourselves, in our ability, in our babies? And why is that important? What if the experience of birth and new motherhood was an extension of the thought patterns created during pregnancy? What if the confidence you find and can nurture in yourself could be bottled and poured over you in those sleepless, confusing first days as a mother?

If you are holding this book you are clearly open to discovering more magic. And to do that you need to take responsibility for, and ownership of, the process you are in; this is essential not only for birth, but also in life.

Looking ahead now to your birth, keep the outcome in mind; and remember ~whether you have an orgasmic water birth or a Caesarean is ultimately not the point. The point is:

- Did you feel you had a say in the decisions being made?
- Were you treated with kindness and respect?
- Did you feel like the most important person in the room?

If you want to be able to say yes to each of these questions, then you will need to take a very active role and lead the process. Take charge and lead the process you are in rather then follow when it comes to all the decisions you make about how to best care for yourself and your baby.

Take a deep breath.

Pause.

Exhale.

Say out loud: 'My care provider is not the person best equipped to make all the decisions regarding my pregnancy and birth.'

Take a deep breath.

Pause.

Exhale.

Say out loud: "I am the best person to make all the necessary decisions about my pregnancy and birth."

Come back and repeat this exercise as many times as you need over the coming months. Reclaiming your power is not going to happen in an instant.

If being a leader is not your natural way, then this is your opportunity to learn!

Here are six simple ways to get started.

1. Choose responsibility instead of blame

Two people in the same company heard that within a few months their company would be downsizing with massive employee cuts. The first person became anxious, wondered why these things always happened to her and started telling her friends the world was out to get her, that she was about to lose her job, and that there was nothing she could do about it. The second person realized there was probably a better job out there for her anyway, so started watching the job classifieds, polishing up her CV and taking more friends in the industry out to lunch to see what the other prospects were out there.

Both got made redundant.

Who do you think walked away from that situation feeling more positive and confident about the future? Don't sit and wait for the outcome you fear. Do your best to avoid it in the first place, and be prepared for it so it doesn't blindside you.

> "I got what I wanted and prepared for, a natural unmedicated birth. No one could do for me, but me."
>
> Laura, first baby, USA/Singapore

2. Control what you can

What happens when you get scared? Do you tend to be paralyzed and spend a lot of time wondering 'what if'? Or do you get proactive and take the reins to control what you can in the situation?

> "I'm proudest of taking control of the birth of my second son. Even through all the warnings and (hospitals and nurses saying) "well that's not our procedure", I was empowered ... I had the birth story I wanted. I love telling the story of his birth."
>
> Dao, second baby, America/Singapore

Sitting in the fear is as useful as invoking our inner victim to come out and play. Instead, if we choose to use the fear to get proactive, to take responsibility, to respond to the situation, we invoke our inner hero. Which archetype would you rather have playing a primary role on the journey to parenthood?

You control:

- The care provider you choose
- The tests you decide to take
- The care you take of your body
- The care you take of your mind and emotions
- The food you eat
- The level of stress you allow/consume

- The images you take in about birth
- The stories you take in about birth
- The books you read during pregnancy
- The type of birth preparation class you select
- The amount of time you spend preparing yourself
- The location you chose for your birth

This list can go on and on, and I invite you to add to it yourself.

3. Find positive role models

We benefit from positive role models in all areas of life.

If I was preparing to launch a startup I wouldn't seek advice from someone who described the experience as horrific, who said they would never do that again and advised staying as an employee in a company. I would go to the person who did a fabulous job of a business launch, and it would be even better if that someone had had challenges to work with that got them thinking more creatively and was prepared to speak openly about all the learning rather than the setbacks – someone who appreciated and enjoyed the journey for what it was. The same approach applies to birth: find someone who had a fabulous experience of becoming a mother and learn all you can from her.

Use caution when using the same primary care provider (PCP), the same hospital, and making decisions in the same way as your friends who ended up with episiotomies, Caesareans, babies in the neonatal intensive care unit and postnatal depression.

If there is no one in your immediate circle, then widen it to find the right people. They do exist. Join a mums' group that has a shared philosophy of positive birth. Work with a professional counselor to practice constructive self-talk.

Read inspiring birth stories on LoveBasedBirth.com and on many other websites. I have included a list of my favorites at the back of this book.

4. Invest in your primary relationship

We often get so busy in our lives that we completely forget to take time to communicate effectively with our partners. Sharing feelings, thoughts, concerns, and fears, and learning to listen to each other, are essential during this time of change.

One of the things my husband and I often use is: "What I feel like saying…" (WIFL). We use it as a simple but powerful way to become present to each other. One of us starts and the other listens, without interrupting; then the other person has a turn. It allows the feelings of whatever is going on to be acknowledged and heard so they aren't unconsciously distracting us from being present.

For example, we both get home from work and one of us had just left a demanding client and the other is just out of a stressful meeting with a potential investor. We want to be present together and with whatever is going on at home, but our feelings and minds are still focused on what we said and felt in our meetings. We often do a WIFL when we sit down at the table for dinner; it only takes a few minutes and will often lead to more connection and understanding in our conversations.

A WIFL goes something like this…

Red: "What I feel like saying is… 'I feel… about… and it..' "That's what I feel like saying, Ross, what do you feel like saying?"

Ross: "Thank you. What I feel like saying is… 'I feel… about… and it…' "

Red: "Thanks for sharing."

The partner who's not talking simply witnesses and listens, doesn't react, interrupt, or try to fix anything. This can be tricky, because it is so natural to jump in and start problem solving or giving our opinion. Sharing our feelings in this way is practice in being vulnerable, leading to more connection.

Another classic example is sex. While a "quickie" can be often therapeutic and serve some needs, great sex is about connection and presence. For me if we haven't connected through our conversations and aired the feelings we might be experiencing, our love-making feels disconnected. Sexual intimacy can guide us back to a place of more communication and sharing.

I love Brené Brown's book *Daring Greatly*; in it she says, ""Vulnerability is the core, the heart, the center, of meaningful human experiences." I couldn't agree more!

PARTNERS: Don't underestimate the importance of your role and presence during pregnancy. As everything begins to change for her, she will want you more than ever. That wanting might look and feel different than it did before but I promise you it is there like a fierce flame. She wants your attention, presence and gentle reassurance. Let her cry and wipe her tears, tell her she is doing an amazing job, how beautiful her changing body is, go to bed at the same time as her at least a few times a week. Ask how she is feeling and listen to the response. Put your phone aside, look at her before you look at your phone in the morning. Generally, do your part to support her to feel like the incredible magic genie, goddess, wonder woman that she is. Remember you are also teaching your little baby about relating, love and partnership while he/she is in the womb.

5. Recognize the quality of your self-talk

How often do you get caught up in a negative self-talk commentary your mind creates for you?

Women often tell me that, while pregnant, they communicate with their babies through thought. They don't feel the need to say things like "I love you" aloud because they know their baby gets the message when they think the thought. In my own pregnancy, I also felt the ease of this silent dialogue. But at times I wondered if my baby was listening to ALL my thoughts.

In the process of writing this book, self-doubt has often come up: "Who do I think I am writing a book? Why would anyone want to hear what I have to say?" It's my old friend unworthiness sneaking back in. We would have a chat, and I'd have to remind myself: I am a creative, intelligent, beautiful woman, and I am making a difference in the world. That feeling is so much more in line with what I want my baby to feel coming from its mother.

Am I successful every day? All the time? No. But that is not the point. We are not going for perfection, after all that doesn't even exist and sounds very stressful to attempt to achieve. However, having another person inhabit your body is great motivation for becoming more aware of the state of your thoughts.

6. How many chemicals are a part of your daily life?

Look through your bathroom and kitchen cupboards, and throw out all the body and cleaning products whose labels feature words like parabens, sodium lauryl sulfate and sodium laureth sulfate, phthalates, triclosan, talc, dyes, and fragrance, to name a few. Cleaning products can be replaced with vinegar, baking soda, coconut oil, essential oil and other natural ingredients that are gentle on the environment, on you and on your new baby.

Swap body products like shampoo, deodorant, and moisturizers with chemical-free versions and get used to reading labels during pregnancy. If it says "all natural", don't take it at face value. Read the label, and learn what it all means.

Do

- Ask yourself:
  - Are you a follower or a leader?
  - How often do you take responsibility, as opposed to playing the blame game?
  - What do you do when you are scared, or feel out of your depth or over your head?
  - Are you a generally positive person or a worst-case scenario player?
- Make a list of what you can control in this process.
- Find positive role models.
- Invest time in your primary relationship. How often do you share your fears and vulnerabilities with each other?
- Start noticing the quality of your self-talk.
- Explore and reduce your chemical load.

CHAPTER 3

....

TIPS – Building Your Team

*"Don't be satisfied with stories, how things have gone with others.
Unfold your own myth."*

Rumi

Part of being a midwife means hearing many birth stories. At a party, in a meeting, at the grocery store, women are always telling me their stories. I don't ask for them, they just come out as soon as someone introduces me as a midwife.

The experience of birth sticks with women. I have had women in their seventies recounting to me exactly what the nurse or doctor said to them during their birth or recalling specific details of how they were treated. We are all walking stories. What will the story of your baby's birth be?

I have spent years exploring what accounts for the differences between women's experiences of birth. What explains the strong opposites on the pain/pleasure wheel; the vast range of difference between the traumatic stories – the "it was the worst day of my life" stories – and the stories of triumph, magic, love and celebration – the "it was the most incredible thing I have ever done" stories? Is it purely luck? Genes? Karma? Yes, sprinkles of fairy luck dust always help. But there is much more to it than that.

The first step in the TIPS formula is team building. Life is a team sport and pregnancy, birth and parenting are no different. Did you have a big wedding? If so, I bet you didn't do it all on your own. Wedding planners, florists, caterers, DJ, MC, dress designer/maker, personal trainer may well have helped; while you had locations to scout, bridesmaids to pick, and a honeymoon to plan.

Imagine doing everything yourself? Think for a minute how it would have changed your experience of the months leading up to the big day and then the big day itself.

There is not only 'one way' to get married just like there is no 'one way' to give birth. I got married with three friends, barefoot in the park, one sunny Saturday in Singapore, after I'd finished teaching my birth preparation class. That sunny Saturday was our 'second' wedding: the first had been planned for about a month earlier but on that morning I was called to a birth. I had a special day welcoming little Oliver into the world, alongside his parents and four brothers and sisters, while my partner drank the champagne with our friends.

However, with birth, there is no easy way out of "let's just plan a picnic in the park", or "sorry, we need to cancel today because something important has come up." Your body is going to move forward regardless if it's the day you had in mind or not, or whether you feel ready or not, or whether you finished your birth preparations. In birth there is no backing out.

I was having a conversation recently with an entrepreneur friend who told me that many Formula One drivers have similar level of skill, so what sets the winners apart from the others is their team. After the mechanical team has set up the car, what plays a big part in the outcome is how fast and efficiently the support team changes the tires, refuels, gets the correct amount of air into the tires, and does all the rest of what they do to get the car back out into the race.

That sounded exactly like birth to me: having a willing team on the side-lines gently encouraging you not only on the day itself, but also in the months and weeks leading up to the event, keeping the environment free of obstacles, and the driver positive and well nourished makes all the difference.

Start building your support team early, but if you are reading this and expecting your baby to arrive in the next couple of weeks, you still have time to evaluate who is on your team. However, the earlier you begin, the more opportunity you give yourself to prepare on all the levels you need to: mentally, emotionally, spiritually, and physically.

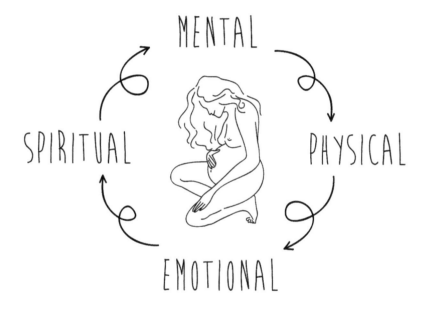

"You've totally got this and you don't even know it! And it needs to be team work, both with your partner (who obviously needs to be totally on board,) but also your wider Team Birth. Have people around you who are positive and awesome and not going to stress you out. You can actively shape your birth, visualise it, practice for it – almost train for it, if you will. You don't have to just sit there and hope for the birth lottery to come good and you get a good birth, you have the chance to take ownership of it."
Nicky, first baby, UK/Singapore

When planning your team, remember to think of the period after the baby arrives. The fourth trimester, your "baby moon", is one of the most important trimesters in which to have a good team in place.

Who is on my team?

Your team can be hired professionals, as well as carefully chosen friends or family members. They might fall into the following categories or you might have a completely different set:

- Birth support/doula

- Nutrition – are you eating as well as you could be?

- Movement/exercise: walking friends, a yoga teacher, a swimming friend, a prenatal exercise class in the park or at the local community center, prenatal yoga classes or other prenatal fitness programs

- Relaxation/stress management: who is helping you (to learn) to relax and unwind? It could be a relaxation track you find online, a deep breathing video on YouTube, a meditation circle, or a walking group

- Alternative health: who can you turn to for advice on natural remedies, so you don't need to reach straight for pharmaceuticals for common complaints like coughs and colds, nausea, indigestion, sleeplessness, restless legs, etc.

- Birth preparation classes: find an independent educator and not a hospital-based educator. Check out hypnobirthing, Lamaze, the Bradley method, Love Based Birth, and sign up for whatever resonates the most with you. There are also great online classes if you don't have any good classes in your area, for example Love Based Birth, check the resources at the back of the book.

- Breastfeeding: who will support you once you're home?

- Self-care: who will cook for you and take charge of the house for those first few weeks?

The professionals on your team might include:

- Midwife

- Doula

- Yoga teacher

- Naturopath

- Nutritionist

- Body worker (osteopath, biodynamic craniosacral therapist, chiropractor)

- Masseuse

- Independent birth preparation teacher

- Postnatal doula

- Breastfeeding counselor

Who you need for your team depends on where you are giving birth. For example, if you are giving birth at home, you will most likely be working with a midwife. Many midwives advise on nutrition, natural remedies for common complaints, breastfeeding, and on the general health of you and your baby through pregnancy and for the first month after birth. You might be lucky and find one midwife who checks a lot of these boxes.

If you are following a medical model – birthing in a hospital with an obstetrician – but want a natural birth, you will want to bring others with a holistic focus onto your team.

Birth is also often compared to running a marathon. Waiting until a few weeks before race day to begin training is not going to set you up for the best experience of the race or give you the best result. Consider how you can train to be at your best physically, mentally and emotionally before then. You might hire a coach, masseuse, running partner, nutritionist, yoga instructor, or anyone else who can add value to your preparation. You might make a few playlists – sounds/music/affirmations to keep your spirits high. Planning, preparing, exploring, and building your support team will help you to experience deeper levels of acceptance and love in how you relate to the outcome, regardless of what it is – an orgasmic water birth or a planned Caesarean section.

CASE STUDY: Calling the shots

I worked with an influential young woman who happened to live in a palace. Because of her position, there was a lot pressure on her to have her baby in a "traditional" way – meaning following the mainstream medical model. But she knew what she wanted and she wasn't going to settle for anything else. She wanted to own the process and make all the decisions. She brought in professionals who could support her vision, including me, all the way from another country. She hired me to work with her during her pregnancy, preparing for the birth and then accompanying her during the birth, to remind her that what she was doing was completely normal and within her grasp. She wanted her baby to be born gently in the water; she wanted dim lights; she wanted to breathe her baby out; she didn't want her baby to be taken away but to stay with her, with the cord intact. At her insistence, the hospital installed dimming lights in the birth room, and brought in a tub and connected to the hot water system. They had never seen anything like this and neither had anyone in the state where she lived.

And she did exactly what she set out to do. After the birth, the chief obstetrician of the country in question, who had been attending, told me, "I have attended more than 10,000 births, but I have never seen anything like that. She was so calm! She didn't scream once. How did you do that together"?

She had overcome family, cultural, religious and medical norms to do what she felt intuitively was right for her and her baby.

·······
Do
·······

- Start to think about what you want your baby's birth story to be.

- Start planning your support team. The earlier you get people on your team who are encouraging you towards your goals, the better!

- Spend time with women/couples who loved their experience of pregnancy and birth, and find out who was on their support team.

- Decide what you want and make those preferences known to the people who will be handling that aspect of your birth.

- If people on your team are not willing, able or trained to respect your wishes look for team members who can do so.

Note: Popular midwives and doulas get booked up early so you might want to engage them first.

CHAPTER 4

TIPS – *The Role Of Intuition*

"Our deepest fear is not that we are inadequate.
Our deepest fear is that we are powerful beyond measure.
It is our Light, not our Darkness, that most frightens us."
Marianne Williamson, author

The second step in the TIPS formula is Intuition: finding it, trusting it, following it. Intuition is a special magical power that we all have, and with a little practice and openness, it can easily be developed.

Back in my days traveling with the circus, I quickly learned how to tune into my intuition because if I hadn't, I wouldn't have survived. I was Fool the Guesser: I guessed people's ages, weights, and birthday months. If I was wrong, they would win a small soft toy. I was brilliant at setting up nice displays, but at the guessing I was... *terrible* – and just waiting to be fired.

However, I was amazed at how quickly that shifted. After several weeks of hundreds of people coming to my stand, I began to tune in to how to read these people, into how heavy they were. Within several months, I was drawing large crowds and had such a blast teasing them and getting them to strut their stuff, making the crowds laugh. It wouldn't be unusual to have someone on my scales that was hitting the 300-pound mark. My estimate had to be accurate to within three pounds if I was to avoid giving out a soft toy. There was no smoke and mirrors or underground weighing scales to rely on, just my intuition.

Me: "Mmm... 287!... Ok, Get on the scales and let's check... 288? Bingo! Who's next?"

The crowd loved it! They thought I had magical powers and I did in a way, I had a developed intuition. Now, many years later, I look back on that time and I can see how that was the start of me trusting my intuition and myself more – something that has served me well as a woman and as a midwife.

What is intuition?

Science has proven that intuition has an anatomical location in the body. We have a "backup brain" in our solar plexus – the middle of the body, the epicenter of nerve activity. It turns out that our "gut instincts' really are nerve signals that guide much of what we do throughout our lives. This gut instinct is our intuition, our inner compass that quietly directs us.

Why is intuition so essential during pregnancy?

Your ability to sense what is right for you and your baby is key to parenting, and remember: parenting starts long before birth. You are the best person to know what is right for you and your baby in every circumstance. If your intuition is enabled you won't have to analyze which path is the right one; you will be able to feel it, to sense it. Accessing, trusting, and responding to your senses will make a lot of the decisions much easier: which care provider to choose, the location for the birth, whether you need that routine ultrasound or test, when it is time to go to the hospital or birth center.

One of my yoga teachers often says during class, "Follow your intuition, not your neighbor." She loves to remind us how important it is to not let the ego lead towards an injury, but rather to let the connection with the body, and what your muscles and ligaments are saying, be the guide. It's the same during pregnancy, birth, and parenting. Whatever your neighbor is doing may not be what is good for you.

There is a saying, "a mother's intuition is the strongest force in the universe." I agree! I have seen it played out hundreds of times. So why can't we always hear it?

The role of fear

Many things can inhibit our ability to sense and to feel, and fear is usually at the root of it. Fear causes constriction, or tightening in the body, that limits our ability to develop, use, or feel our senses fully. This limitation can lead to disconnection. If we're not careful, time passes – nine months, for example – and there we are, stuck in worry and fear, completely limiting our ability to take a leading role in the process of pregnancy and birth.

> "Every time I feel unsure about something, I just go with my gut. I try not to listen to what everyone else says, as everyone says something different. So that has honestly helped me throughout pregnancy, births and as a mother."
> Jasmine, Singapore

Fear is very loud. It shouts at us; intuition on the other hand, whispers. Women often ask me, "How do I know whether I am hearing my intuition or my fear?" I answer, "How loud is what you are hearing?"

If we take the time to explore our fears, we find they have a silver lining: they propel us into action and into taking responsibility for reducing the possibility of a negative outcome. Take a look at the following example.

Your primary care provider (PCP) tells you on multiple occasions that your baby is "very big".

Do you:

- get very nervous?

- tell all your friends?

- start having nightmares about the birth?

- tell your baby to stop growing or start starving yourself for fear the baby will get bigger?

- book your induction or Caesarean?

Or do you

- ask your PCP questions to understand the full picture of what he/she is saying?

- find out what having a 'very big' baby means, what the risk factors are, and how can you avoid them?

- tell them you would like to re-evaluate at the following appointment and, in the meantime,

  - evaluate your diet: do you have more sugars (simple and complex) than you need? Do you have enough wholefoods, vegetables, and proteins? Maybe you can find someone for your team who can help you with this.

  - make exercise and movement a priority: you know your baby will be the perfect size for your birth, and you want to be as fit and healthy as you can for the birth.

- trust and affirm to your baby and your body that they know exactly what they are doing?

- consider a second opinion?

Can you see the difference with the two approaches? We will come back to exploring and working with fear guides in Chapter 8.

Your inner compass

Here is a pregnancy quote I love: "You are stronger, more intuitive and more flexible than you have ever been before!"

How true! I cannot encourage you enough to spend time tuning in, focusing on your baby and on your body to begin hearing your quiet inner compass.

> "I feel much more connected to my intuition now than before my pregnancy. It brought me trust in the pregnancy and birth processes and brings me faith in life as a new mother and in general."
> Marie, first baby, France/Singapore

When you are at your doctor's appointment, turn your inner compass on. When you are taking hospital tours, turn it on. When you're wondering if your baby is growing well, turn it on. When you're deciding whether to take any of the tests you're offered, turn it on! You and your baby will be glad you did!

Next time you see your care provider, ask yourself whether this person sees pregnancy and birth as normal and natural, or as a medical condition to be managed? Ask yourself for the answers to all of your questions. I promise you, they are sitting right there.

We will look in more depth at how to strengthen your intuition in Chapter 7.

Do

- Begin cultivating an awareness of your bodily sensations – notice if you are tense and tight or receptive and open.

- Keep a noticing journal – note down when you hear your intuition and follow it. What happened? What was the outcome?

CHAPTER 5

TIPS – *Partnership Health Care*

*"In 2017 whether or not a woman will have a Caesarean is not
dependent on the risk factors she presents with;
but which door she walks thru."*
Dr Neel Shah MD, MPP, Assistant Professor at Harvard Medical School

The third essential step in the TIPS formula is Partnership health care. The couples who have the best experiences of birth do this very well. I can't emphasize the importance of this step enough. Don't skip it, don't miss it.

How many of you married the first available, handsome, well-groomed, fit, successful person you met? I didn't think so. Me either. I kissed a *lot* of frogs. There are too many other factors that make for a good match, right?

That's why we date: we get to know someone, find out if they are on the same page as us, whether they share our same dreams, aspirations, and view on life. Only then do we take the next steps of commitment.

I would like to suggest that there is no difference when it comes to choosing a primary care practitioner (PCP) for your birth. No, I am not suggesting you date your potential care providers, but *do* interview them, get used to asking open-ended questions, shop around, and find a good fit for you. You are looking for a care provider who will support you as an individual, encourage you to have questions and opinions, and who is willing to partner with you for a good outcome.

Depending on where you live, your PCP could be a midwife, an obstetrician, a family physician or GP. You can fast track making a shortlist of care providers to interview by asking mothers in your area who they used and what their experiences were. If you don't know any new mums, then look for a new mum breastfeeding group or a place where new mums meet up, and go there and ask questions.

Above all, don't just go to the same PCP as your friends if they all had Caesareans and negative experiences of birth – the chances are that you will have the same experience.

If you find yourself making justifications for your PCP like:

- S/he didn't answer my questions, but that's because s/he was in a hurry.

- S/he was very rough in the examination, but I guess that is the way it happens.

- We don't have the same view, but s/he is very experienced at what s/he does.

- I don't agree with her/his approach, but s/he is very nice.

... *please* re-evaluate; it is time to move on. Your birth is too important for both you and your baby to settle for someone who isn't a good match, for someone you are with because they are a family friend, because they "delivered" you, or because they go to your church.

Confidence is key to this process. If your PCP is not helping you to find more of it, if you're not leaving your appointment feeling more confident and relaxed then when you went in, it is a sign that something is wrong. You are not with the PCP that is right for you.

I am often surprised how common it is for women to treat changing their PCP like a divorce. "But they have been there for me during a difficult pre-conception time. How can I just leave them now?" Let's be honest. Your care provider will remember your birth for five minutes, whereas you will remember it for a lifetime. It is your responsibility to make it your experience rather than someone else's.

"[I am proudest of] not being submissive and taking charge of my own body and my birth experience. For some it may seem like too much work, risky or a hassle, but I felt it actually made things a lot easier down the road."
Freji, second baby, Indonesia/Singapore

A concern that comes up a lot in this conversation is, 'When is it too late to change my PCP?" or "I am already 28/32/37 weeks, isn't it too late now?" In my opinion, it is never too late or too early to make any big decisions in life.

CASE STUDY: It's never too late
I recently worked with a woman who was planning a vaginal birth after a Caesarean (VBAC) and had taken the trouble to find one of the most supportive doctors in the city – but he hadn't mentioned to her that he would be on holiday on her due date.

When she turned up at the hospital in labor, she found a stand-in junior doctor. He wasn't interested in her birth preferences and expected her to spend her labor lying on her back with the heart rate monitor strapped on. She wasn't allowed to walk or eat, or even drink water, because he thought she was too "high risk".

There was no way she was prepared to follow his instructions, so she checked herself out of the hospital and went straight to the office of another VBAC-supportive doctor in town who agreed to take her on, and she had the birth she imagined later that day.

Which type of primary care practitioner?

There are two types of PCP:

1. Opinion-based, active management, high-intervention practitioner

2. Evidence-based, expectant management, low-intervention practitioner

The opinion-based or active management PCP is likely to answer questions with an attitude of 'Who are you to question me? Where did *you* go to medical school?' Their responses may include

- Your baby is looking too big, I'm not sure it will fit out of the birth canal.

- VBAC is not a safe option to consider.

- No episiotomy might be OK for Western women, but all Asian women need one.

Or the ultimate:

- "You stick to being the patient and let me be the doctor."

With responses like to these, you will know they are a high-intervention practitioner. Please do not make it your responsibility to change his/her views on birth or hope you'll be the one with whom they see the light. It's not worth it. Switch care providers.

By not following well-documented best care practices, this active-management PCP would likely put you and your baby at higher risk of other interventions, like expecting you to lie on your back for the birth or be hooked to up to an IV drip and monitors during labor, or not observing your wish to delay the clamping of your baby's cord.

If, on the other hand if they listen to and invite your questions, encourage you to have opinions and to participate actively in your care, treat you as an individual, give you options and respect your decisions; then you are with an evidence-based, expectant management, low-intervention PCP.

Remember, don't make assumptions about your PCP: the range of experience is vast as is the types of practice they offer. Just because they have a nice office or work at the newest, fanciest hospital does not mean their practice protocols will be up to date.

How to interview a PCP

Ask opened-ended questions. These start with "who", "what", "when", "where", "how" and "what". As they articulate their responses, you will gain a much better idea of their philosophy. However, asking each of these suggested questions in a single visit will probably not feel appropriate, so I recommend asking the first three questions on the next page. They will give you a good idea for this practitioners philosophy.

Turn on your intuition and be open to needing only to hear the response to the first question to get a good idea if the PCP a good fit or not. The subconscious, intuitive, self works fast.

> "I changed my gynaecologist in week 32. After having a planned necessary Caesarean for my first child, it was very important to me to deliver my second child naturally. Despite telling her my wish for a VBAC [vaginal birth after Caesarean] from the beginning, she only told me in week 32 she was unwilling to support my wish because she considered me high risk. (I changed doctors and) I was very happy with the provider I moved to and had my successful VBAC!"
> Jeanne, second baby, France/Singapore

If there is potential to continue the relationship, you will begin to relax in your chair and feel comfortable, or at least experience a certain amount of ease – that's the sign you're looking for. Maybe save the rest of the questions for the next visit, unless, of course, time permits and it feels in the flow.

Your approach

Take a few good deep breaths in the waiting room. Straighten your back, roll back your shoulders, and feel that your feet are on the ground. Remind yourself not to interview aggressively or defensively, as such an approach will not elicit a positive response, no matter who the practitioner is. Do whatever you need to do to express neutral, open, confident curiosity.

Questions on these three topics will give you a clear idea of what sort of a practitioner you have in front of you.

1. In what circumstances would you feel it is necessary to cut an **episiotomy?**

    Examples of opinion-based/active management replies:

    - birth is taking too long

    - first-time mum

    - Asian mums

    - to use the vacuum

    - baby is too big

    - to avoid a tear

    Then "Out of every 200 births, how many times do you use an episiotomy for …(insert the reason given)?"

2. In what instances do you find **induction** is necessary for healthy mums and babies?

    Examples of opinion-based/active management replies:

    - big babies

    - reaching 40 weeks

    - reaching 41 weeks

- cord around the neck

- mother doesn't want to wait any more

3. What **positions** do you support women to birth in besides on their back?

   Examples of opinion-based/active management replies:

   - you must be on your back so I can see/manage your birth

   - we use stirrups

   - usually always on the back but we can see how it goes for you

If time permits, these are other good questions relating to birth:

- What do you think about women eating and drinking in labor?

- At what point, once labor starts, do you expect me to come to the hospital?

- What if my waters open as a first sign of labor: how much time do you give after that for labor to begin naturally if my baby and I are healthy at that time?

- How do you feel about me having support people, like a doula? How often do you work with doulas?

Examples of opinion-based/active management replies include:

   - it is better not to eat or drink during labor – you won't feel like it anyway

   - it is good to come in as soon as your contractions start or as soon as your waters break – there could be a problem

   - only your husband/mum is allowed in the room – birth should be private.

Also good to know:

- What percentage of your patients give birth without an epidural?

- What is your personal Caesarean section rate? What is the most common reason your patients have surgery?

Remember, some PCPs will have a 80% Caesarean rate and some will have a 2-10% rate. It is your job to find out which is which, to give you and your baby the best chance for the best outcome.

> "[I am proudest] that I wasn't scared when the doctors told me that my baby was 95th percentile large! I knew I would be able to handle birthing my baby. And I am proud that I chose home birthing despite family and friends being worried. I didn't let their fear poison what I intuitively knew was right for me."
> Catherine, first baby, Singapore

Note: You are legally able to accept or decline any procedures offered to you, except in genuine emergency (labor is not an emergency), such as a life or death situation or if you are unconscious, with no next of kin. No decisions can be made about your care unless and until you agree to them.

Do

- Approach selecting a primary care practitioner with great curiosity.

- Be committed to finding an evidence-based, low-intervention practitioner.

- Treat the exploration like an interview process.

- Ask open-ended questions.

- Turn on your intuition at all your appointments.

- Remember you are your baby's and your own best compass.

CHAPTER 6

·····················

TIPS – Making Time For Self-love

"Love is the capacity to take care, to protect, to nourish.
If you are not capable of generating that kind of energy towards
yourself – if you are not capable of taking care of yourself,
of nourishing yourself, of protecting yourself – it is very
difficult to take care of another person."
Thich Nhat Hanh, Buddhist monk and peace activist

The fourth step in the TIPS formula is making time for Self-love.

Pregnancy is a perfect reason to start taking extra good care of yourself. You have more demands on your body so extra nourishment in the form of TLC becomes more of a necessity. You are in a time of major change and transformation, and being extra kind and gentle with yourself is vital for enjoying the process.

Let's not forget the little one, is also immersed in our experiences. During this time of gestation, just as during parenting, it is our responsibility to keep the environment safe, positive and supportive. It is a perfect time to start breathing through discomforts and stresses: this practice will help you immensely in labor, when you are tired and done with working through your birth surges, when you are trying to keep your eyes open with a crying baby, or when your toddler asks "why?" for the thousandth time. You are in training, and putting a priority on self-love now will have benefits for a lifetime.

Self-love comes in many different shapes and forms. A big part of it is slowing down, being a bit gentler with yourself, and not having such a full to-do list every day. Give yourself more room, more permission to do things that feel good rather than things you feel you *should* get done.

Creating more space will also help you in the early days of mothering. I see all the time how challenging it can be for women who have accomplished a lot in life, are very motivated, are at the top of their fields, who carry a lot of responsibility at work – when suddenly everything stops after birth. When they feel like all they have been doing is breastfeeding, and wonder if they have even brushed there teeth. New motherhood is meant to be a blur; that's ok, it's normal. The more you can slow down and give yourself space now, the more it will cushion the shock of the big shift in your perceived efficiency in the coming months, and the easier it will be for you to take the slow, repetitive nature of motherhood in your stride.

Slowing down, reducing stress and taking time to pamper yourself, for example, have many health benefits and will help prevent pre-term labor, strengthen your immune system, and increase your connection and confidence.

I learned a lot about self-love by having a nervous breakdown. Early burn-out is something common in midwifery, sadly, because so often it attracts women who love to care for others and, in doing so, forget about themselves. Hitting rock bottom and needing literally to crawl my way out has revolutionized the way I practice midwifery. I take on fewer clients and fewer births; I charge more for my time because I respect it more; I make sure to always do something good for myself after a birth, especially a hard one; and I take time to do my own rituals for processing the experience – that's a must.

I believe that as care providers we have a responsibility to the families we work with not to carry around our own emotional baggage. When we do, we can have a negative effect on the way labor progresses and on the outcome of the birth for that mum and baby. I encourage you; if you are looking for a midwife or a doula to support you, to ask about how many births they take on at a time. Ask what they do to relax outside of work and how they care for themselves. And then choose someone who values themselves as much as they value you.

Here are some ideas to care for yourself and your growing baby over the coming months. I know you can come up with your own big list, so please do!

> "Someone told me not be afraid to do things that make you feel happy and alive. Pregnancy is not an illness. Don't listen to what others think you should and shouldn't do because only you know what your body is capable of. You don't have to stay on a couch the whole time!"
>
> Filza, second baby, Malaysia/Singapore

Bubble wrap

Commit to building a positivity bubble around yourself that only allows in people, conversations and experiences that build your confidence and make you feel good.

I am amazed at how beautiful, glowing pregnant women seem to be a green light for people to start projecting their own fears, horror stories and traumas onto.

When someone wants to share a birth story with you that starts something like, "it was the worst day of my life", give yourself permission to stop them right there. Prepare ahead and practice a few kind statements that you can use so it is easy to get them out, just in case you get frozen in the moment:

- "Thanks for wanting to share your experience. I'd like to have my own baby first, and we can swap stories after my birth."

- "Let me stop you there. Let's have this conversation again in a few months."

I promise you that there is already more than enough negativity in the media, on the news and all over the internet without you having to listen to your neighbors' and taxi drivers' stories too. Everyone has a story to tell, and it is important to them to tell it. However, this is not the time for you to help them process their difficult experience of birth.

Fill your bubble with positive stories and images of birth. Don't watch birth videos on YouTube, as you never know what you will find that doesn't serve building your positive birth space. You are not being naïve; you know birth doesn't always go according to plan. There are things in your mind that you don't even remember are there, that you have seen at some point in your life, depicting birth as horrific – time to create new pathways and be the author of your own thinking.

Only let in what helps to boost your confidence, making you feel, "I can do this! I was made for this!"

> "The best advice I was given was early in pregnancy: turn off the TV birth shows! Although I had some level of fascination of having an inside look into what is typically a very private event, I learned that those types of shows serve up inaccurate, medically-biased labour and birth information that reinforce ideas of fear and pain. In late pregnancy: trust the wisdom of your baby. He knows how to birth himself and it is essential to his emerging problem solving and learning."
> Stacey Lee, first baby, South Africa/Singapore

I guarantee you there are many good, positive stories of birth available if you know where to look. It is like restaurants – if you have a fabulous meal and get fabulous service, you are probably going to tell two people about it. If, on the other hand, you have a terrible meal with crap service, you will probably tell ten people – this is the nature of our psyches.

"My partner was awesome! He did loads of things that I'm so grateful for, but the biggest was that he was absolutely prepared to put aside his (and my own) preconceived notions about birth and embraced hypnobirthing, love-based birth and home birth. This is radically different from his family and upbringing, but he became such a passionate advocate for it. He was also a gatekeeper for me, if people were starting tell to a negative birth story or question or birthing choices, he was great at just politely but firmly shutting that down. Definitely, don't listen to negative birth stories! Shut yourself off from that. I find it amazing that people love to share horrific birth stories when you're pregnant."
Nicky, first baby, UK/Singapore

Active relaxation

Practicing active relaxation every day is important both for your long-term health and your baby's. Unplugging from all your devices and spending time focusing on your breath, heightening your senses, learning to spot tension in your body, and then knowing how to let it go – all these are essential not only for the birth, but also for experiencing more freedom and pleasure in life.

Here is a simple exercise you can do now; I call it a body scan.

Sit back in your chair and close your eyes.

Breathe in, sending the air deep into your belly so it expands outward.

The next time you breathe in, count 1-2-3, and feel your belly expand.

As you exhale, breathe and feel your belly soften as you count 1-2-3-4-5-6.

Repeat this breathing for several rounds and then while continuing to breathe into your belly, get curious about where you feel tension in your body.

- Is your forehead tight?

- Are you squinting your eyes closed?

- Is your jaw clenched?

- What is happening with your shoulders – are they somewhere up by your ears or are they relaxing down your back?

- What are your hands doing? Are they soft and open?

- What about your belly muscles? Clenching or holding?

- Butt? Vagina? Thighs? Feet?

As you notice the tension, let it go as you breathe out. This is good to do throughout the day and when you lie down at night before going to sleep. There are more ideas for relaxation in the next chapter.

> "(During my labor) I was able to block out most surrounding stimuli and be in my own zone. When the pain got very intense, my doula and my husband started to breathe, almost like chanting with me. It was wonderful and helped immensely. I felt so supported, and it helped me to deal with the pain and to find a rhythm for breathing."
> Teresa, third baby, Singapore

Sexual pleasure and orgasm

Unfortunately, many couples get told that they shouldn't engage in love-making or penetration sex during pregnancy. This is an opinion-based statement not based on any research.

Note: There can be medical indications for pelvic rest, which means no penetration or orgasm. These include placenta previa (or low-lying placenta), open waters, or active signs of pre-term labor. However, this is a small percentage of typical, healthy pregnant women.

I have heard it all, from the range of bizarre advice given by PCPs, to the common and often peculiar fears couples express about sex during pregnancy, for example:

- You will poke your baby in the eye.

- You may turn your baby into a sex fiend.

- It will cause a miscarriage.

- Your baby will be embarrassed.

- Your baby shouldn't be 'participating' in such an act.

- It will start premature labor.

These are all myths based on other people's guilt and shame about their sexuality. Don't take them on board. Your baby is well protected in its private little cosmos; you are not going to poke it or harm it in any way. Your body is also too perfectly designed for something as natural as sexual pleasure and orgasm to trigger labor in your second trimester.

Oxytocin, the hormone that is released when you experience pleasure – which peaks at orgasm – is known as the hormone of love, safety and trust. Science shows that whatever hormones the mother releases cross over to the baby. I would rather my baby felt the sense of love from oxytocin than the anxiety from adrenaline and other stress hormones! Bathing in oxytocin helps the nervous system to relax, and I can imagine the growing baby loves to feel his parents loving each other.

Sex during pregnancy can be challenging because of the changing physical, emotional, and mental landscape we find ourselves in.

The changing hormones of pregnancy affect every woman differently; some will experience an increased sex drive, and some will find their drive lowers. Sexual pleasure and orgasm, whether you are pleasuring yourself or you are with your partner, are a healthy part of a normal pregnancy. Sex is a good way for you to relax, de-stress, and connect to yourself and to your partner. As your body changes, you will need to experiment with different positions to accommodate your growing belly and to feel comfortable. Many couples start to prefer a side-by-side position.

> **Note:** A woman's changing body affects every partner differently. I know many women whose partners lose sexual desire during pregnancy. They may feel intimidated or frightened by the wiggling baby, or generally view her body in a different way. That's OK, too. Remember, you don't need someone else to release oxytocin!

The important thing is for you to keep the communication open and stay in touch with what feels right for you both.

Caring for your body

Body brushing

Body brushing is a great habit at any time in life, and pregnancy is a good reason to get into the habit if you are not already doing it.

Good circulation is very important during pregnancy. By the time you reach 28 weeks, your blood volume has doubled. Your arteries and veins are fuller than normal, placing more strain on them. Dry brushing helps to keep the blood moving and to reduce the chance of getting spider veins and varicosities. It also moves lymph and fluid and helps support the immune system.

Always brush towards the heart – up your legs, up your arms, down your chest and upper back, up your bum and lower back, up your belly. I also like the act of simply taking that extra time in the morning. Rather than rushing into the shower and into the day, make time for slow morning rituals.

Here's how to get the best out of body-brushing.

- Buy a brush made of natural fibers. I like the long handle ones to get those hard-to-reach areas of the back.

- Spend two or three minutes loving and brushing your skin before getting into the shower each morning.

- Be gentle around your tummy – your stretching skin might be more sensitive to the brush fibers.

Epsom salts baths

Make it a priority to get into the bath once a week during pregnancy. This is a self-love practice that promotes the wellbeing of your physical and emotional body. The water helps ease any aches and pains, and the soak relaxes the nervous system and melts away stress hormones. Both will help you get a good night's sleep.

Why is adding Epsom salts a good idea? Because Epsom salts are pure mineral compounds of magnesium and sulfate. Stress quickly eats up the body's magnesium stores, increasing the flow of adrenaline and other stress hormones, so it is important to replenish it. Magnesium is important for many functions in the body, including reducing inflammation and helping muscle and nerve function. It also helps in the production of serotonin, which is a neurotransmitter that plays an important role in balancing the mood and can ease headaches. Sulfates draw toxins out of the body and help it to absorb nutrients.

Adding Epsom salts means bath time will help boost your immune system to keep you healthy and active, as well as reduce aches and pains. If you have an active cough or cold or flu, then consider bumping up your Epsom salts soak to three times a week instead of only once.

If you don't have a bathtub, you can also use a bucket to soak your feet and legs.

Here's how to make the most of bath time:

- Put your devices aside.

- Light a couple of candles and maybe put on your favorite relaxation music.

- Use one packet of Epsom salts (roughly 50 grams).

- Don't use any other soaps or put oils in the water.

- Keep a big glass of water beside you.

- Stay in for at least 20 minutes.

- The water should be warm, but not so hot that you heat up your core body temperature.

Prenatal yoga

Prenatal yoga is one of my favorite and most recommended movement practices during pregnancy. I have seen in women who practice regularly (at least three times a week) have an increased capacity to manage the intensity of labor. Yoga builds strength and focus, and at the same time cultivates surrender and relaxation.

One of my prenatal teachers loves to get us into squats. She keeps us there for a minute, and then we release and go back into it for another minute. She does this in rounds, and as our legs begin to shake, she reminds us to find our breath, to find movement to help keep our focus. "This is your practice contraction," she says, "find your breath, get comfortable with the intensity, soften into it."

Prenatal yoga will help you to sleep better, to have a stronger body, to become calmer and more relaxed, and to connect with your body and your baby.

> "The best advice I received was to walk a lot and to cultivate a prenatal yoga practice – especially squats and becoming familiar with my own sounds. Also, connecting to my growing baby through meditation and self-belly massage. I believe these things helped me with birth and to develop a deeper connection to the process of becoming a mamma."
>
> Tonia, first and second baby, Canada/India

Pregnancy is a great opportunity to start a gentle practice if you haven't before. Be sure to sign up for a prenatal class with an experienced prenatal teacher. The benefits will be lifelong, especially if you keep it up after the baby comes.

> **Note:** whether you are a skilled practitioner or a beginner, your pregnant body has different abilities and requirements that we want to respect and accommodate. Be kind and gentle with yourself, go slowly when you need, be open to wanting a very different practice then you did pre-pregnancy. Tell your instructor that you are expecting at the beginning of class – no hot yoga or deep twists during pregnancy.

Here are some more ideas for self-love and to ensure you're staying on the oxytocin side of life!

- Eat loads of fresh fruit and vegetables.

- Get midwifery care!

- Listen to music you love.

- Take plenty of naps.

- Get a good water purifier.

- Drink lots of water!

- Get craniosacral, chiropractic, or osteopathic care.

- Dance.

- Meditate.

- Connect with your friends.

- Go on dates with your life partner.

- Get massaged frequently – as a minimum once a month. Learn to do self-massage as well.

- Take time off.

- Do things that make you feel good!

- Get creative.

- Sing.

- Go for walks.

- Spend money on experiences, not things – massage, bodywork, yoga, dates, etc.

Pregnancy is not a process that is happening to you. It is a process that one way or another you have invited. Relax into it, enjoy it, treasure it. Be kinder to yourself than you have ever been. Give yourself permission to stay in bed if that's what you need today. Your body is growing a human and needs rest.

Do

- Make time for self-love and self-care

- Start building a positivity bubble around yourself – no more birth stories unless they are positive.

- Go to Love Based Birth and watch the birth videos there, which have been carefully selected to help you boost your confidence.

- Take weekly baths with Epsom salts.

- Start dry body brushing.

- Active relaxation: use the body scan technique while in bed, before you go to sleep.

- Consider joining a prenatal yoga class

CHAPTER 7

The VAGUS Model

"Birth isn't something we suffer but something
we actively do and exult in!"
Sheila Kitzinger, author, birth activist

How can we start to quiet the noise of the thinking brain – the neocortex – so we can begin to develop a stronger relationship with our intuition?

While connecting to our intuition is simple, it is also an ongoing process that needs effort and repetition. For me, it is basically a process of creating the environment and the opportunities to connect inwards, to notice what comes up, and then to trust my intuition to guide what I do next.

I have created the simple tools of the VAGUS model that give us that opportunity to connect inward. These tools have helped me and many other expectant parents to get more connected as we progress towards parenthood.

V – Visualization

A – Affirmation

G – Guided Meditation

U – Understanding the Mind Body Connection

S – Sound Breathing

The VAGUS practices will automatically begin to highlight where we are disconnected. While exploring our fears is important, we don't need to understand them – the dark side, or the shadows – fully; rather, we can dive into the light and see how it begins to chase the shadows out of hiding.

We will all resonate differently with each of these practices, depending on whether we are more visually, auditorily, or sensorily inclined. The only way to know what works best for you is to play with each one! Whenever you are visualizing and affirming, pay attention to what comes up; these are the juicy bits.

Breathing

The single most important tool to become very familiar with is your breath. Using the breath to cope during times of uncertainty or discomfort, to bring focus and the capacity to cope, is something you probably do without even realising it. Have you ever noticed how when you stub your toe on the edge of the couch, it feels much more intense if you hold your breath? It is safe to assume birth is the same. Breath is the bridge into each one of the VAGUS practices, the bridge that leads us back to our intuitive selves. Start by practicing breathing into your belly: slow inhale, – belly expands; slow exhale, – belly relaxes.

> "My breath was my ultimate companion on the birth journey. From all the years of practice with yoga and meditation, this companionship came easy to me, and I am extremely grateful. Focusing on long, slow breaths allowed me to face the intensity of the surges and to breathe through them. The breath also helped me to breathe my baby down, to breathe her into my hands. As the intensity of the surges increased, I started using sound breathing, and this was absolutely paramount in my experience. The low sounds helped me to stay extremely present, while at the same time relaxed my cervix/vagina/pelvic floor due to the mirror effect. Also, the sounds carried me through the surges."
>
> Amber, first baby, USA/Singapore

Visualizations

Positive visualization is a tool that is used by top athletes and professionals in many different fields. Recently, I watched the movie *Rush*, about Formula One winner James Hunt. In the movie, he rehearses for the race by simulating driving the course in his mind. He would lie back on his couch, close his eyes, and imagine driving through each twist and turn of the racetrack, practicing the gear changes, leaning his body with each of the turns right and left.

Albert Einstein says, "Imagination is more important than knowledge."

See it, feel it, breathe it… your mind does not know the difference between real and imagined. And visualizing will create muscle memory – on 'race day' James Hunt had already done each turn of the course many times, so it was fluid and automatic. What if we looked at birth the same way?

But what does 'positive birth' look like? Filling ourselves with positive images of birth during pregnancy is essential, but where do we 'input' these images from? I created a gallery of birth videos on Love Based Birth that I invite you to watch and you can scroll through at your leisure. It is much safer then cruising YouTube with the prospect of encountering unwanted surprises of images that don't serve your positive image bank. Typing 'gentle water birth' in your search is not going to ensure you see something positive, because everyone has a different idea of what that means.

As we start filling up the positive image bank, we also need to recognize all the negative images we might have stored – All those movies with emergency birth scenes, the women screaming, everyone shouting and scrambling about, sirens, alarms, bells and whistles. And what about all the 'horror' stories you have heard from your friends, relatives and other people in your community?

It is important to acknowledge that they are all sitting there in your memory bank. And that's OK – we can let them be just what they are: sensationalist TV or the experience of people who didn't have all the information you have, who probably didn't put time into developing their team, building partnerships with care givers, cultivating intuition, and taking responsibility of the process and the outcome like you are. You can let it all be and make a resolution not to fill up this image bank any further. Turn off all the shows that are not building your confidence – *One Born Every Minute* and other reality birth shows really aren't serving you.

These are common visualizations we use during pregnancy:

- your baby floating in the optimal birth position;

- your cervix opening (only practice this visualization after 36/37 weeks); and

- seeing and feeling your ideal birth

The more we give our minds the opportunity to be playful, to imagine and wander and explore like they did so easily when we were six years old, the better. Exercising this part of your brain will make it easier for it to come up with something helpful to keep you present and focused during labor to cope with each birth wave.

Note: When using visualizations it is best to *feel* yourself in the scene rather than *watching* yourself in the scene.

"I kept repeating 'relax' and 'open' to myself and visualized flowers opening. This helped during earlier contractions. Listening to my husband do a relaxation visualization we had practiced helped during hard labor, when I was spiralling and focusing too much on the pain. He brought me back to something familiar and refocused me away from the contractions."
Catherine, first baby, Singapore

Women who have spent time visualizing during pregnancy have shared all sorts of stories with me of the mental images that arrived spontaneously during labor to help them through each surge.

> "I was somewhere in active labor. I had my eyes closed and was breathing with the surge when out of nowhere a man on a yellow surfboard appeared. As I rode my birthing wave so did he. I watched as he rode up one side of the wave and then down the other. I knew if I kept my focus on him, I would manage each surge, and I did."

> "With each surge, my mind played out a scene where I was walking down a staircase into a basement. I don't know what I was looking for or what I was doing there, but if I went with that scene with every surge, it was very manageable. I didn't even need to use sound during transition. I just kept feeling myself walking down each of those steps."

> "For both my births, I felt the surge like steam coming under the doors of the room I was in. During each surge my mind would work to push the steam back under the door and if I could stay on top of that steam with my mind, the surges were very manageable."

Each of those women had used visualization during pregnancy, but none of them had practiced that specific visualization. Their brains were stimulated and playful, and they were receptive to going along with whatever came up because of the practice they had done during their pregnancy.

Affirmations

Saying, writing, and listening to affirmations are all great ways to connect with the positive feeling of your expected outcome.

The key with affirmations is that they shouldn't be used to cover up fear like a Band-Aid, as in "I have a strong fear of having a Caesarean but I know I should just have faith that it will all be fine so I'll just say this affirmation every day: 'My body is capable of giving birth naturally.'"

It's lovely to have that intention, but until you address the fear, it won't go away and will instead loom large like the white elephant in the room. Address fears by turning them into action and responsibility (the ability to respond), and then use affirmations to settle positivity into your cells. Taking action in this example might mean finding out the top reasons that Caesareans occur and how to avoid them, finding out your PCP's Caesarean rate to establish whether they are as committed as you are to avoiding an unnecessary one. We will look at working with fears more in the next chapter, and at Caesareans in more detail in the last chapter.

> "My doula wanted me to have a phrase or affirmation that I connected with…I was guided to 'every surge (contraction) brings me closer to meeting my baby'. That connected with me – and I remember smiling and thinking that affirmation during the second stage of labor…yes, I was smiling!"
>
> Lori, third baby, Vietnam/Singapore

Here are some examples of affirmations for pregnancy and birth:

- My body is nourishing the child I am carrying beautifully.

- My choices throughout this pregnancy are based on love, not fear.

- I decide how I feel during pregnancy, and I choose to feel vibrant, healthy and strong.

- I trust my body.

- I surrender my birthing over to my baby and my body.

- The power and intensity of my surges cannot be stronger than me, because they are me.

- I breathe deep and slow to relax my muscles, making it easier for my uterus to work.

- My baby's size is perfect for my body.

- Each surge brings my baby closer to me.

'I am' statements are very powerful, I encourage you to find three words that resonate and feel good when you say and feel them in an 'I am' statement. For example:

> I am strong, powerful, safe, loved, supported, healthy, vibrant, connected …

Breathe the affirmation deep in your belly and then release it with your breath as you soften and relax.

Tips for using affirmations

1. Write your own, using words that resonate for you.

2. When it comes to writing affirmations, they need to have all eight of these Ps:

   - Present tense

   - Positive

   - Personal

   - Precise

   - Powerful

   - Private

   - Plausible

   - Persistent

Each of these Ps are important and here is an example of why: There was a woman who wanted to attract a wonderful man into her life. She wrote down all of the attributes she wanted him to have: funny, passionate, smart, rich – the list went on. Well, soon she met an incredible man who ticked all the boxes! And his name was Rich and he didn't have any money. Be as precise as possible. Even saying financially rich wouldn't have been clear enough. What if he was cheap, and not generous with his money? Be as clear as you can with what you are asking for, always, in every area of life.

3. Your subconscious will be able to work with the affirmations best when they are in your native language.

4. Choose three or four to work with for pregnancy and three or four to work with for birth.

5. Write them out and put them somewhere where you will see them many times throughout the day – maybe on your bathroom mirror or on your refrigerator.

On the Love Based Birth website you will find many more affirmations and ways to use them.

Guided meditation

Guided meditation, also refered to as guided relaxation, is a wonderful way to connect with yourself and with your breath, and to enter a state of relaxation without having to think about what to do. You can simply take a comfortable seat, or lie down and be guided.

Guided meditation can be done by listening to an audio track, or to someone reading a script to you or by talking you through it on an impromptu basis, either in a group or one to one. Today there are many free audios you can download, and there are also apps like Mindspace, Mind the Bump, iHypno and others.

Tips for using guided meditations

1. No one track will suit every woman, so explore to find ones that resonates with you.

2. A track in your native language is ideal.

3. Putting on a track several times a week will help to reduce your stress level and help you to become more focused.

4. Listen at a time when you can actively relax and find your breath rather than have it playing in the background while you cook or do other activities.

5. If you have trouble sleeping at night, if you are tossing and turning and feeling uncomfortable, this is also a good time to put on a relaxation track.

6. Have your partner record a track for you. There is a sample script to use on the Love Based Birth website. Modify it to suit you: be playful, have fun, push out your boundaries. Embrace the opportunity: there may not be many other times in your life when you get such an opportunity!

Pick a guided track you love to listen to and can imagine using for labor. Listening to it frequently will build up relaxation body memory, so that when you play it in labor your shoulders will automatically soften and your breath will deepen. Your body will already have that memory. Do the same with several music tracks.

"I felt connected to my intuition during my pregnancy. Meditation really helped and still does help for me to hear that inner voice a little more clearly. Sometimes I do ignore it and most always I feel disappointed that I didn't speak up."
Tonia first and second baby, Canada/India

Understanding the mind–body connection

The mind does not know the difference between imagination and reality. I invite you to keep hold of this fact and think about it throughout the day today.

Consider the example of the last time you watched an intense thriller movie. You were sitting on the edge of your seat, heart racing, palms sweaty, and if someone had come up behind you and startled you, it would have been enough to make you jump and possibly scream.

Why? Your mind was in the scene and stimulating your automatic nervous system to produce stress hormones like adrenaline to prepare you for the fight-or-flight response, in case you had to run like hell or beat up the intruder. Yet there you were, completely safe in your house, on your couch, with someone you love and eating great popcorn. Your mind didn't register that you were completely safe and that the scene was all made up and had nothing to do with you.

Science is now proving that our entire body chemistry changes depending on whether we are thinking of a sunset or thinking of a lemon. Each of our thoughts causes chemical responses in the body and those chemicals create the picture of our reality.

Grantly Dick-Read, an English obstetrician, came up with the Fear, Tension, Pain theory which he discusses in detail in his book *Childbirth Without Fear*, first published in 1942. He explains how fear causes us to tense up, that it's the tension that causes us to experience pain.

Many women enter the labor room today feeling fearful about what will happen, on the basis of all the scary stories they have heard, and all the dramas they have watched. The fear may not be based on any reality but the body doesn't know that, so it responds with the defense that keeps us safe: the flight-or-fight response. "Get me out of here!"

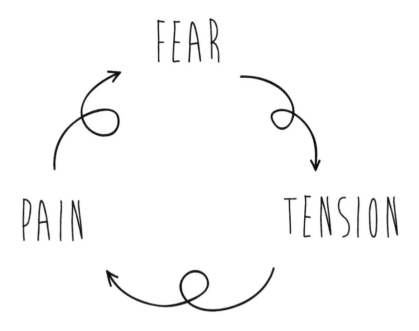

FEAR

PAIN　　　　　　　TENSION

Muscles tighten, surges become more painful (remember, the uterus is a muscle), the increased pain causes more tension, the tension causes labor to slow and now all the common interventions are called into the birthing process.

You are given an intravenous drip with synthetic oxytocin (Pitocin) to get labor going again. Now, with the drip in place, you need to stay in bed, usually on your back (the most unnatural way to work with labor), and the surges are no longer your body's but are pharmaceutically induced, strong and back to back, and your body isn't producing its natural pain-killer, endorphins. It is too much to bear and you ask for an epidural. Once that is in place, you also need a urine catheter because your legs are numb so you can no longer walk to the bathroom. Now you also have a blood pressure cuff on your arm, and a heart rate monitor strapped to your belly to monitor the baby. You can't feel the urge to push even though the baby is ready to come out, so vacuum or forceps are used for the delivery.

This is a very common scenario, and is called a "cascade of interventions".

Another common outcome of this cascade is that the baby gets tired. The contractions are unnatural and coming too fast. Mum can't move, rock and sway to help the baby figure its way out. The heart rate monitor picks up the baby's distress and a Caesarean is called. Everyone breathes a sigh of relief that the doctor was there to save the day. But how do we know it wasn't all the intervention and stress that caused the distress in the first place?

> **Note:** I am not anti-epidural or anti-intervention – I have been the first person at a birth to put my hand up to ask for an epidural for the mother, because I don't believe birth is about suffering. If it feels like suffering we need to do something to change it. I do, however, strongly believe in the importance of being well informed. Many women who I interact with have no idea that an epidural means all the other interventions will be there hand-in-hand with it. It is marketed as a miraculous savior and left at that.(See more about the potential negative side effects of epidurals in Chapter 12.)

Understanding how our thoughts create our reality is key to more freedom and joy in life, as well as in birth. Are we the master or the slave of our minds? Let's do the work required in advance so that when we walk into the labor room, our nervous system is relaxed. Relaxed because we are informed, prepared and confident in our body's ability to handle whatever is coming up.

This is the central point for me as an educator. I want every woman on the planet to do her work long *before* labor, so that her mind has less chance of overtaking and sabotaging what is meant to be a magical, beautiful, joyful meeting between her and her baby.

That is why we are here together, learning how to get off the fear, tension, pain wheel and instead on the love, confidence, and relaxation wheel. The more love space we create from working with our fears, the more confidence we will feel, and the more we will be able to stay relaxed and let our bodies do what they naturally want to do. Open.

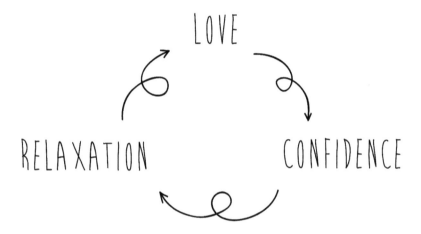

"I avoided discussed my birth plan with people who I felt would question it; I only wanted positivity around me and the birth, and I wanted to stay out of my head (other people's opinions can sink me into thinking, thinking, thinking) and into my body and energy channels, including my intuition, the Higher."
Caroline, second baby, UK/Singapore

Sound breathing

The single most powerful tool to use during labor is sound breathing. Hundreds of women have told me after birth, regardless of how many different strategies they practiced before, that when things got rough, sound was their key focal point, guiding them over the waves.

I first discovered the term "sound breathing" while working in a water birth center in Goa, India, with a fabulous German midwife named Corina. An opera singer who was interested in the sounds women make during birth had come to the center to learn. She sat outside the birth room listening for many births to the sounds the women were making and from that she designed a program for women during pregnancy, gathering each week to play with making sounds in preparation for birth.

Those days at the birth center were magical! It didn't matter where we were in the building, the entire place was echoing with the most amazing, deep sounds that automatically gave you goosebumps and a strong feeling of connection.

The rate of women transferring to the hospital was extremely low at that birth center – well under 5%. And during my time there – about 6 months and about 40 births – not once did we transfer a woman because she wanted an epidural. I know that has a lot to do with the sound breathing women were using to cope with labor's intensity.

Sound is not only for birth, as I previously thought. Practice making deep sounds – the types that vibrate around in your body. Make the vowel sounds O, U, A like this every day during pregnancy and it will help keep tensions and anxieties at bay. It is a wonderful addition to your self-care routine.

Here's why: The vagus nerve is the 10th cranial nerve, the longest nerve in the body. It is nearly as thick as the spinal cord and it is the captain of the parasympathetic nervous system, which is the control center for harmony and balance in the body. This nerve runs down from your head and touches each one of your organs, controlling many functions like heart rate and digestion. Science shows that people with tight, contracted, and lacking-tone vagus nerves often have corresponding symptoms of tightness, anxiety, stress, and depression in the body.

Science now suggests that stimulating the vagus nerve plays a role in alleviating stress and tension. This stimulation can lower the production of stress hormones such as adrenaline and catecholamine, and increase the release of pleasure hormones like oxytocin and endorphins.

Put your hand up if you want a relaxed vagus nerve and more harmony and balance in the body. Yes please!

How do we reach inside and stimulate the vagus nerve? Sound vibration. We can use sound that causes the vagus nerve to micro-shake – vibrating, elongating, expanding, and toning. These powerful yet subtle movements begin to bring back its tone and shift us from the sympathetic flight-or-fight mode to the parasympathetic mode – the harmony and balance strand of the automatic nervous system. This is exactly what we need in the intense moments of labor. I see all the time how using low, tonal sounds can immediately move a distressed women in labor into a focused state.

> "During my pregnancy, I listened to meditation tracks on a daily basis; I trained my mind with affirmations that I wrote on colourful posters that cover our bedroom walls; and I practiced breathing and sound breathing (low sounds) on a daily basis. By the time of the birth, I no longer needed to listen to the meditation tracks or look at my posters as I knew them by heart. I used the hypno-birthing breathing techniques and I used the visualisation of a blooming flower during the opening phase and a picture of my cat with wide open legs during the birthing phase."
> Marie, first baby, France/Singapore

Other benefits of using sound during labor

Ina May Gaskin, quite possibly the world's most famous midwife, suggests the lips, throat and jaw mirror the vulva, vagina and cervix. I couldn't agree more. They are both midline structures after all, and it make sense that whatever is happening above is also happening below.

The other day I was talking to a postnatal rehabilitation physiotherapist who attended one of my talks on preparing the perineum for birth. When we started talking about this mirror effect she said, "Yes! We see that all the time; often women with a tight perineum and pelvic floor issues also have very clenched jaws. When we work on the perineum we always work with helping the woman to relax her jaw."

Opening the throat opens the path for the baby. Using deep sound to open and relax the throat when labor intensifies will help that last bit of cervix to melt around baby's head with ease. It is also a great focal point for the mind as you travel into the sound you are making. Because it stimulates the vagus nerve, it will also help you to feel more relaxed and calm during the most intense part of labor.

"Using sound helped me to channel and focus on the low tones and that sent a vibration throughout the body. I was not using the throat but used my diaphragm to create the low tones and that helped to calm and relax my mind. I needed the vibrations running in my body to mask the pain from the surges. The surges seemed to be more manageable. I was not afraid."
Kasturi, first baby, India/Singapore

The sounds need to be open – think of the vowels AOU – rather than the more closed sounds of I and E, which have the opposite effect, constricting and tightening the throat and jaw.

With a history of anxiety and panic attacks, I would generally describe myself as someone with a sensitive nervous system; I have used sound with very positive results. I came across the use of sound again while in training programs with the Indian mystic Sadhguru. He describes the benefits of chanting Aum daily around twenty-one times and goes into detail about how to get the sound to vibrate in the body.

> "Sound breathing helped a lot...it felt natural to do it and almost like I needed to, otherwise there was no other way to release all the tension. It helped me through each contraction by focusing on the pitch being low, focusing on the volume not being too loud...it basically gave me another focus, so almost like meditating through it. My sound was more like an oooooo, rather than an oooommm."
> Dao, second baby, Singapore

It made sense to me. After I started practicing using sound daily, it wasn't long before I felt the benefits. My system was changing: I was more relaxed, less anxious; more confident and better able to cope with the usual ups and downs that life brings.

Using sound to clear energy channels in the body is an ancient practice. In traditional Hatha Yoga, sound vibrations are used to clear the seven chakras (centers of spiritual power in the body). The sounds chanted are:

Lam – chakra 1 (root)

Vam – chakra 2 (sacral)

Ram – chakra 3 (solar plexus)

Yam – chakra 4 (heart)

Ham – chakra 5 (throat)

Om – chakra 6 (third eye/brow)

Om – chakra 7 (crown)

Remember Julie Andrews singing "do, re, mi" in *The Sound of Music* with the von Trapp chldren? This exercise is taught to pitch notes and sing in tune, and now we know it can also help us *live* in tune.

So in the moment of birth we can use sound to create a positive physiological change in the body, and using sound consistently over a period of time we can change the flexibility of the vagus nerve to create more harmony and balance in the body.

Do

- Stimulate your creativity

- Spend time building your positive visual collection of birth.

- Try visualizing your baby in the best position, and seeing and feeling your ideal birth. (more on optimal position in chapter 16)

- Create three or four affirmations to work with during pregnancy, and three or four to work with during the birth.

- Create three 'I am' statements

- Find one or more guided meditation tracks to help you relax at the end of the day.

- Start to notice how your body reacts to where your mind goes.

- Notice when you are holding tension in your jaw and consciously release it.

- Play with, and get familiar with, making low sounds; try to make sounds that vibrate in your body.

CHAPTER 8

·····················

Working With Fear Guides

*"They who do not fear darkness have
learned to light their own candle."*
Dodinsky, author, *In the Garden of Thoughts*

Fear is not bad; it is normal. If you feel fearful of some aspect of pregnancy, labor, birth or parenting, there is nothing wrong with you. You are not being melodramatic; you are normal –considering all the scary stories you have heard about birth for the last few decades, or sensationalized births you have seen online or in movies.

The practice we want to establish here is noticing the fear when it pops up, but not letting it completely control our decision making and our lives. Fear in the present moment keeps us alive. It stimulates the fight-or-flight response that kicks in to get us out of danger. When we are flooded with adrenaline and stress hormones, we can run faster than usual and for longer, or we can quickly whip our hand away from the fire. We move in and out of aspects of fight of flight all day.

Fear of the future is also normal, especially when that future is so unknown – something so big that we have never experienced before, like pregnancy, birth and parenting. There is a blessing in the fear; it is guiding you into unknown areas so you can address them, become familiar with them, make them OK, and get your mind/body back into a safety zone.

The most common fears I hear are

- Caesarean

- Pain

- Tearing

- Not being able to 'do it'

- Dying

- Something being wrong with the baby

- The baby being too big

The reason why it is so essential to identify and then process your fears of pregnancy and birth is because if you don't, they will dominate you. They will dictate which care providers you pick, what tests you do, the decisions you make, and, ultimately, the type of birth you will have. Until you become friends with them, they hold too much power over you, and they will have too much attraction power – your mind loves to be able to say, "I told you so".

"Because I've experienced birth many times, I've learned that my body has a voice separate to my conscious mind. That voice is shrill and panicked and believes the worst, when I'm in heavy labour my body screams at me "I'm dying! Escape! Get me out of here!" But I have learned that I can discipline my thoughts and stop that voice and almost step outside of myself to speak to myself from a calm place and focus on the joy and euphoria ahead. I spend a lot of time allowing the part of my mind that I can control to still the voice of panic or fear. When I do this it is so empowering, it feels like I can do anything when I get all of the voices and feelings aligned."

Tammy twelfth baby, Australia/Singapore

The Five-step Process

I use this five-step process to work with fears:

1. Name it: write the fear down and talk about it with your partner, midwife, doula.

2. Get informed: what increases the likelihood of this fear becoming a reality? What are the risk factors? What are the myths? Gathering information increases your power and puts you in the driver's seat.

3. Action steps for prevention: list all the steps you are taking to avoid this outcome.

4. Management: if that fear or outcome does become reality, how will you make the best of the situation? How can you set yourself up to find grace and ease in the situation?

5. Affirm: you have done your work, but that doesn't mean it may never pop up again. If it does, use affirmations, visualizations, or talk to the fear: "I am noticing you, but you have no place here anymore. I have done all of my work and am putting my trust in God/nature/my body/the Divine."

First step: what are my fears?

Get a piece of paper and write these four words down on the side of the page:

- Pregnancy
- Labour
- Birth
- Parenting

Now write down everything that you are worried about or afraid of – all of your fears, no matter how big or small. Be honest with yourself.

Take your time and come back to this list if and when new things pop up over the coming weeks and months. The more you get out here, the clearer you will be in addressing your fears as you move forward. It is important for your partner to do this same exercise and for you to discuss it together.

Here's a worked example of how to explore each item on your list.

1. Name it: fear of tearing or episiotomy (a surgery the PCP does to cut the vagina and make it bigger for baby to come out)

2. Get informed: take a good birth preparation class to understand when cutting an episiotomy is necessary, whether it is better to tear or be cut (a natural tear of the muscle will heal better than a cut because tears are jagged and have more surface area for healing compared to the straight line of a cut, which often results in more scar tissue. The World Health Organization recommends episiotomy only for emergency procedures.); and learn what increases your risk of tearing:

   - poor tissue integrity

   - birth position (flat on back, legs in stirrups)

   - hard pushing and tension while baby is crowning

   - being rushed/directive pushing

   - PCP who has little experience with natural birth

   - size and position of baby's head

   Consider whether tearing is as bad as you imagine: the perineum is made to tear a little if it needs to for birth. It heals incredibly quickly. It is like the inside of your mouth. Remember those times when you bite it accidentally and it starts to bleed? You feel as if you've bitten a piece out of it, but then your tongue is poking around later that day and, like magic, there is already a new layer of skin. The same thing happens in the vagina. I stitch less now for a minor tear and prefer instead to teach the woman to care for it naturally because I see how well it heals on its own.

3. Action steps for prevention: these are practical things you can do to prepare yourself.

   - Great nutrition: eat healthy fats and reduce sugars.

   - Exercise and stay active.

   - Take 20–40 mg of zinc daily.

   - Choose a PCP wisely – someone who only does episiotomies in an emergency and understands natural birth, and allows for position of choice

   - Prepare the perineum with Epi-no (a pelvic floor trainer) and perineal massage.

   - Practice relaxation and breathing (take a good birth preparation class)

   - Learn about natural positions for birthing (lying on your side, on hands and knees).

   - Learn what "mother-led" pushing means and put it on your birth plan.

   - Learn to actively relax, to soften the perineum. Notice when you are holding tension in it and when you are relaxing it.

   - Strengthen your pelvic floor.

   - Watch the video on Love Based Birth, "How to prepare the perineum for birth".

4. Management: discover how you can support your body to heal easily if you do have a tear.

   - Prepare ingredients or order in supplies for sitz baths. (more in chapter 25)

   - Arrange for home support for the first few weeks, giving you more rest and recovery time.

- Buy breathable/natural maternity pads (less plastic and perfume will mean faster and more efficient healing).

5. Affirm: repeat these statements to yourself regularly.

- My body and baby know how to work together to give birth.

- My tissues stretch beautifully around my baby's head.

- I feel my baby moving gently down and take the time I need to let birth unfold at its own pace.

- My body is made for birth.

- My baby is a perfect size for me to birth gently.

Once you go through this process with each of the fears on your list, you will most likely see a degree of repetition coming up in your action column. For example, you might see movement and exercise, paying attention to nutrition, choice of PCP coming up frequently – those areas that repeat need special attention.

See how your fears, when you are conscious of them, can become your guides to a better birth. Embrace their wisdom, and see where they are directing you.

> "I was afraid that something could happen to my baby while in the womb that would make an early delivery necessary, and also that during birth (for both my children) that something bad could happen to me or them. I worked with my midwife with both fears and became confident in both pregnancies that I was growing a healthy child and that I was supporting them as much as I could by doing all that I could to make sure I was healthy and they were comfortable inside me. While the fears didn't disappear, I was so well prepared with the help of my midwife that I forgot about it during labor and was totally focused on my boys and was so looking forward to finally meet them."
> Andrea, first and second baby, Germany/Singapore

....
Do
....

- Begin embracing your fear guides.

- Write out all your fears about pregnancy, labour, birth and parenting. Share them with your partner and have him/her do the same

- Use the five-step method to turn those fears in positive action.

CHAPTER 9

....

Parenting Before Birth

"Babies in the womb are alert, aware, and attentive to activities involving voice, touch, and music; babies benefit from these activities by forming stronger relationships with their parents and their parents with them, resulting in better attachments and better birthing experiences. These babies tend to show precocious development of speech, fine and gross motor performance, better emotional self-regulation, and better cognitive processing. These are the gifts and rewards of active parenting."

Dr David Chamberlain PhD, Psychologist, teacher,
and pioneer in the new field of Prenatal Psychology

Modern-day obstetric practices became common during a time when we were in the dark ages of understanding fetal development and life in the womb. That's how we ended up with twilight sleep (a drug cocktail of morphine and scopolamine) that knocked mums out for days, pulling the baby out with forceps, hanging the baby upside down and smacking it on the bum to make it cry at birth, routine separation of mother and baby, and early circumcision without pain medication, to name but a few of the horrors.

Those practices are perhaps more understandable during a period when our understanding was limited to the concept that newborns were incapable of feeling pain or having experiences, but not today.

Thanks to technology, our understanding has completely shifted in the last ten to twenty years, and we now have a comprehensive picture of babies in the womb. The private cosmos your baby is growing in is no longer a dark mysterious place; we know babies are interacting and learning in their pre-birth environment. This understanding gives us a greater responsibility as parents and health care practitioners to do our best to ensure that the womb environment, the baby's first school, is the best that it can be.

By the second trimester, babies have all these senses working for them:

- Touch: feeling touch and reaching out to touch. They love interaction: there are some beautiful videos of twins interacting in the womb.

- Thermal: sensing hot and cold – you may notice that your baby reacts if you eat or drink something cold.

- Sensing pain: grimacing and crying in the womb during invasive procedures.

- Hearing: as they can hear from the beginning of the second trimester, they know your voice well by the time they are born.

- Balance, gravity, and spatial orientation: babies have been seen to fight off needles during amniocentesis at 7–12 weeks, protecting their space and showing aggression to the invader. They also seem to be able to distinguish above, below, front/back, and left/right.

- Smell: your amniotic fluid will smell differently from that of your friends, because you have different diets. This memory of smell will affect their food preferences in the future.

- Taste: all the taste buds are developed in utero. The baby learns about food by swallowing amniotic fluid, which will taste of what you have eaten and begin to set a familiar food palate.

- Mouthing, sucking and licking: it's not about food, but about exploration – the fetus will do all of these to explore textures of soft/hard, and the contours of objects. By 13 weeks they are licking their fingers and toes, and the placenta, and exploring all corners of the womb.

- Vision: babies are seeing by six months and notice how the light filters through your belly. They love to study and watch their beautiful placenta smiling down on them.

- Concepts and social relationships: graceful movements in the womb show self-expression and communication of needs and interests. (Twins have been seen on ultrasounds hitting, kicking, kissing, and playing together.) Womb babies know whether they are wanted based on discerning the feel of those around them.

All that sensing and exploration is going on in this exact moment inside your body!

(This information is adapted from the work of Rudolf Steiner and David Chamberlain – see the further resources at the back of the book.)

Some not so good news

Experts in the field of perinatal psychology and pediatrics are discussing how life in the womb is more vulnerable now than ever before. We are carrying higher levels of stress, are exposed to more radiation, and have more interventions during pregnancy: ultrasounds, overprescribed antibiotics, and other medications. We are consuming genetically modified foods, pesticides, and vegetables grown from depleted soil. We breathe more toxic chemicals from plastics, flame-retardants in our mattresses and couches, and have increasing air pollution – the list is long. Babies in utero today have a far greater exposure than they did even one generation ago; let alone if we consider back to our grandparents or their parents.

At the same time, autism and other neurodevelopmental challenges like ADHD, autoimmune disorders, asthma, allergies and diabetes are skyrocketing. The Center for Disease Control in America states that today one in every 45 children are on the autistic spectrum. It makes sense to ask ourselves how we can safeguard the magical kingdom of our developing babies' environment to the best of our ability.

Science suggests that our parental influence on our children is at its highest during pregnancy. There is no other time in life when you will have as much influence on who your child will become, both physically and emotionally, as you do during pregnancy. Close your eyes take a deep breath. Read that sentence again.

There is no other time in life when you will have as much influence on who your child will become physically and emotionally as you do during pregnancy.

Everything is optional

There is no test, screening or procedure that is mandatory in pregnancy. Every parent should choose what they take or don't take based on having all the relevant information available to make that decision. True informed consent means you have been told about the benefits, the risks and the alternatives. This is where having an aligned PCP is essential. Pregnancy care should not feel like a dictatorship; on the contrary, as PCPs, we are only here to present you with options, including:

- Down syndrome screening
- amniocentesis
- 20-week anomaly scan
- routine ultrasounds
- gestational diabetes screen
- prenatal RhoGAM (a blood therapy recommended in some circumstances)
- prenatal vaccines

Only you know what is best for your child and whether you are someone who feels better with more information or less, whether too much information makes you worry or whether less information does.

For example, Down syndrome screening is known to have a high false positive rate. It is not a diagnostic test, but gives you the likelihood of your baby having a chromosomal condition. That means it is possible to receive a prediction of a strong chance of a Down syndrome baby for one who doesn't have it. I have seen several cases like that: the parents were relieved when their baby was born without Down syndrome, but also upset that they had spent so much time during pregnancy feeling anxious.

No one can make the decision for you, and no decision is right or wrong, especially if you have made it from love rather than fear.

Ultrasounds

As ultrasounds have become more and more popular, they are being used more as entertainment than diagnostic tools. The intensity of their radiation is also getting stronger and stronger, with 3D and 4D imaging now readily available. In medicalized maternal health care systems where midwives are not the leaders in prenatal care, women and babies are exposed to ultrasound at every prenatal visit. It is common for a woman to have had ten to twelve ultrasounds by the time she reaches full term.

By contrast, midwives and many other PCPs use low-tech instruments like their hands and a measuring tape to assess how things are progressing and to identify the baby's position.

Technology doesn't automatically equal better results and it can actually do more harm than good. It has been demonstrated that ultrasound waves heat up tissue and what that heating up does is hard to prove. FDA biomedical engineer Shahram Vaezy states, "Ultrasound can heat tissues slightly, and in some cases, it can also produce very small bubbles in some tissues." If you are anything like me, you will have no interest in unnecessarily risking bubble creation in your baby's tissues. What's more, this heating of the tissues is getting researchers at the University of North Carolina excited about the potential to use ultrasound as a method of male contraception. When applied to the testicles, it lowers sperm count by killing them off.

Disconnection

Another issue I see arising from ultrasounds being done at each prenatal visit is the level of disconnection it creates in mothers. Hundreds of mothers have said to me "But Red, seeing my baby on the screen is how I know it is growing. I find it very reassuring, it helps me connect with my baby."

While I understand that, and I mean no disrespect, I also find it frightening that this need for external validation is becoming so common. Connecting to the intuition is one of the most important gifts for a mother. If we begin to rely on a screen to tell us our babies are OK rather than sensing it, communicating with them, feeling them moving, and feeling these moves getting stronger and growing; how will that affect our confidence as new mothers when we don't have a screen to rely on?

I would like you to consider, until further long-term studies have been done, that the safest routine is to assume less is more during pregnancy. Of course, there are times when ultrasounds are indicated, and then they are wonderful diagnostic tools. However, if we were meant to peer into the womb every five seconds, we would have been designed with a window.

Close your eyes and connect with your baby. If there is something you need to be aware of or to investigate, trust yourself to receive that message.

"I have always been a very intuitive person; coming into pregnancy though, it increased even more. I loved this flowering and gained great confidence with it. Intuition guided me as to what foods to eat, how to nurture my baby, what she needed while growing in utero, how the birth would be, and how to connect to her (before, during and after birth). I had a silent communication with my baby from early on in the pregnancy, and especially during the birth. I feel this connection is what has helped me to find my role as a mother. I've read several books on pregnancy, birth and parenting, and heeded much advice from others, but at the end of the day it is my intuition that has guided me the most beautifully. A mother knows. The more that I can drop into my body, into my heart, into my knowing, the more easily my life flows. Certainly, I feel that having a low-intervention pregnancy (minimal scans) and a zero-intervention birth all helped me significantly to grow my intuition as a new mother."

Amber, first baby, America/Singapore

The best physical environment

We will look in the next chapter at the important points of good nutrition to consider. There are all sorts of clever studies that show that because the baby is smelling and swallowing your uniquely flavored amniotic fluid, it is becoming familiar with tastes and establishing lifelong patterns for food preferences. One of the single most important factors for whether your baby is diabetic in the future might be how you eat during pregnancy.

Reducing chemical exposure as much as possible is also important, and here are some simple ideas for doing so:

- Get familiar with the Clean Fifteen, Dirty Dozen (the list of fruit and vegetables most and least likely to have pesticide residues), and do your best to buy organic for the Dirty Dozen.

- Buy a good vegetable wash that breaks down the pesticide oils covering your fruit and vegetables.

- Get used to reading food labels, but also the labels on all the products you use in your house and on your body.

- Give nail polish and gel nails a rest during pregnancy and breast-feeding.

- Throw out all the chemical soaps, detergents and cleaning supplies in your house. Make your own or buy natural ones. You won't want all this stuff in your house once your little one gets mobile anyway. You'll be amazed what you can do with vinegar and baking soda!

- Don't buy a new couch or mattress during pregnancy, unless it is organic.

The best emotional environment

Will your baby come into a loving, connected world or one that needs to be feared? Will there be time for communication and relaxation, or is it a world where everything is always rushed?

Your baby is not growing in an incubator somewhere, but inside your body and so naturally experiencing what you are experiencing. If we are highly stressed, releasing adrenaline and other stress hormones, with our heart rates increasing, the baby will be experiencing the same thing. If we are releasing feel-good hormones like oxytocin and endorphins, and breathing deep and feeling relaxed, with an easy heart rate, then so will the baby.

The difference between us and them is that we have much more context for everything that we are experiencing than our baby does. We know when we are stressed that it is just because of the movie we are watching or the deadline we are striving to complete at work. The baby, though, is simply experiencing those things without the context. For all they know, you really are being chased by a bear!

It is our responsibility to reduce or buffer the level of stress we expose ourselves to while gestating. If it is possible that just a few minutes of mindful connecting, slowing down and breathing consciously every day could alter the course of your baby's life for the better, who she chooses as a life partner and her other relationships, would that be a good enough reason to do it? Could she simultaneously be giving you the best gift possible by starting you on a course of self-discovery and self-care?

How you can support positive emotional patterns

Your baby is not looking for some sort of perfection, it is looking for you – you being real, fully experiencing and connecting with life. Express your feelings fully; don't keep them bottled up. If you need to cry, cry. Don't allow your body to be an emotional dumping ground.

We are usually taught that emotions such as anger, fear and grief are negative emotions, but in fact they are healthy emotions that serve us well. Anger helps us defend our boundaries; grief helps us to deal with losses, and fear protects us from danger. Fully experiencing your emotions will help you to release them and move back into the light. Illness occurs when we bury and block out our feelings.

Don't deny emotions; truly experience and fill your senses with them, they will move on and so will you. None of us are living on top of a mountain meditating all day. We will naturally have ups and downs. That is normal, this is life.

When you are in an emotional storm, or having a shouting match with your partner, or in the middle of some other stresses, get into the habit of checking in with your baby to say, "It's not about you." Get into the habit of using this phrase, and claiming your emotions as your own. Add something more along the lines of:

- "Mummy is having a hard time today; I am doing my best, so please bear with me."

- "Mummy is processing some feelings today; it is not your fault."

- "I'm feeling sad/angry/hurt/upset and it is not about you. You are loved and wanted."

- "It is not about you; none of it is caused by you. You are loved; you are welcome to be here with me."

- "Your dad and I are working out our differences. This is a normal part of life. Don't worry, you are wanted and loved."

> **Note:** There is no 'perfect'; it doesn't exist. And how terrible would it be to have 'perfect' parents anyways?! Don't worry if you miss a day here or there. Do your best and enjoy it. Stay kind and gentle with yourself and know you are doing the best you can in your given situation.

Tips for communicating with your baby throughout the day

1. Communicate with your little one as if she is right in front of you.

2. Talk to him; he loves to hear your voice.

3. Touch your belly often when you feel kicks and nudges, and give your baby an idea that you are there and listening.

4. Include your baby in your daily activities: "What do you feel like eating?"

5. Pick a song you like and sing it often; your baby will remember it and it will be a great tool for soothing her that you can use after the birth.

6. Play games: your baby might get bored in there and look forward to your acknowledgement. Tap on the spot where he kicks, wait until he responds, and repeat the taps. You will see how quickly he will start to respond and even follow you around your belly.

7. Babies love it when their other parent takes time with them, so at the end of the day, get your partner to acknowledge him by talking to him and rubbing your belly.

8. Have your partner read to the baby.

Dr Thomas Verny, a psychiatrist who founded the Pre and Perinatal Psychology Association of North America, suggests taking daily "fetal love breaks": ten minutes to focus on your breath and visualize your baby – how she is positioned, what she is doing (sleeping, playing with her toes) how she is feeling (playful, sleepy, curious). As you connect with your baby, imagine love and peace filling your belly, and a white light of protection all around it.

Do

- Start thinking of yourself as a parent from today

- Reduce unnecessary chemical exposure.

- Discuss with your PCP limiting the number of ultrasounds for the rest of your pregnancy

- Actively lead on all decisions about which tests feel important to you during pregnancy. Gather the information you need to make informed decisions.

- Communicate with your baby throughout the day, –keeping in mind all the senses he/she is already using.

CHAPTER 10

Nutrition

"Our food should be our medicine and our medicine should be our food."
Hippocrates

What better time to develop healthy food habits than during pregnancy? Eating healthily is important now, not only because you are growing a baby, but because you are also setting up lifelong food preferences for your child. Think colors and include greens, yellows, reds and purples in your daily diet.

You only need about 300 extra calories a day during pregnancy. The idea of "eating for two" isn't accurate. However, if you have a magical super metabolism and you are ravenous, then go for it!

Personally, my food intake nearly tripled in the first trimester. I couldn't believe how hungry I was! I wanted carbs (something I usually rarely eat) but I surrendered and went with it because it made me feel good. I had very little nausea and no vomiting, and I believe a big part of that was because my belly was probably never completely empty.

To combat nausea, you also want to make sure you have enough proteins. Try including things like boiled eggs, nuts and beans, or hummus. I was an egg and Brazil nut fiend, often getting up in the middle of the night to get a handful of Brazil nuts. The other thing that worked for me was potato chips. I bought the better brands, obviously, but boy did I *have* to eat potato chips!

Here are some other ideas to keep nausea at bay:

- Avoid greasy fried foods.

- Eat something small every two hours, ideally a protein and a natural sugar.

- Get a seasickness wristband.

- Don't leave home without a snack in your bag.

- Use aromatic herbs like chamomile or cinnamon.

- Drink peppermint tea.

- Increase electrolytes, try sipping coconut water.

- You may need to stop your vitamin supplements.

- Take ginger in all its forms: ginger root powder capsules, tea, ginger candy chews or lozenges.

- Eat dry foods like crackers.

- Get plenty of fresh air.

- Try meditation

Be kind to yourself. This phase will pass, and until then your body is doing a beautiful job caring for those multiplying cells, regardless of your less-than-perfect diet. I loved the idea of "allowing" in the first trimester: nap when you need to nap; don't judge how you feel. If you don't feel like going to yoga or doing any exercise, so be it. Cry, and feel sad, if you are sad. There is a lot going on in your body! Your hormones are all shifting. Remember, cell nutrition comes in various forms: yes, one form is food, but we also nurture our cells with our thoughts. Surrender to the couch and your potato chips, and trust that this will change again when it needs to.

"The best advice I received during pregnancy was to take better care of myself during my pregnancy by looking after my diet/nutrition for both the baby and myself. I had just passed the horrid first trimester and the nausea and vomiting stopped, however I was still not looking after my diet well despite on having much better appetite than before. The advice/reminder given was like a big wake up that changed not just my nutrition but that of our entire family."

Freji, second baby, Indonesia/Singapore

Once you're back to yourself, a good general guideline when preparing meals is to look at your plate and see that it includes:

- Iron
- Calcium
- Vitamin C
- Protein

Iron

Iron plays an important role in keeping your energy up. Your blood volume has doubled by 28 weeks, and it is natural to see a decline in your blood iron levels around this point. You can ensure it doesn't dip too low by including iron in your diet.

Generally, iron comes from greens and reds: Dates, raisins, pomegranate, beetroot, leafy greens. Good quality free-range eggs are also a good source of iron, as is meat, if you are a meat eater.

Calcium

Calcium is important for strong bones and teeth. Your baby gets most of what it needs by drawing on your body's supplies, so you need to ensure your body's levels are not being depleted. Depletion may not show up for you until menopause, potentially in the form of osteoporosis or losing your teeth.

Forget about drinking a glass of milk a day to meet your calcium needs. Milk is now so pasteurized and homogenized that there is nothing good left in it. Cows today are given too many antibiotics to prevent infections passing into the milk from their wounds, which result from not having enough fresh air and exercise. If you feel you can't live without milk, then please make sure it is organic and, whenever possible, from a known source. Calcium can come from other sources, some of which might surprise you:

- Broccoli
- Kale
- Almonds
- Cheese
- Sardines
- Kefir
- Bok Choy

Do more research to find high-calcium foods. See which of them you like, and ensure they are a part of your daily routine.

Vitamin C

Vitamin C is important for keeping your immune system healthy and happy, and for healthy elimination – yes, pooping! You burn up vitamin C quickly when you are stressed, run down, and living in a polluted environment.

Constipation is considered a 'normal' symptom of pregnancy, because your hormones cause a slowing of movements of the digestive tract.. However, you need to have a bowel movement every day to be in the best of health; if not you are storing toxins and wastes. Getting enough vitamin C in your diet will help you to eliminate daily.

Vitamin C sources include:

- Broccoli
- Kale
- Red/green peppers
- Kiwi
- Oranges
- Guava
- Berries
- Dark leafy greens

Supplements

It is always best to get your nutrients from food first and supplements second, because when we take supplements, we cannot be sure how much the body will actually absorb. I don't think every woman needs to take the same supplements during pregnancy. I prefer to do a dietary evaluation before recommending further supplementation.

The common supplements that you might want to consider include:

- Folate
- A good prenatal combined multivitamin and multimineral
- A probiotic
- Magnesium

- Omegas
- Vitamin C
- Vitamin B
- Vitamin D

The importance of protein in pregnancy

When I think of proteins and pregnancy, I see stabilizing building blocks both for both mother and baby.

For baby

Imagine for a minute growing another human: organs, bones, arms and legs – all that connective tissue and blood – and everything happening without you needing to pay any attention. That is what your body is doing, and it is incredible! It's a clever orchestra of nature supported by the foods you eat.

During the first trimester, protein's amino acids help to deliver nutrients and oxygen to each of the fetus' cells, building your baby's growing bones and muscles. These amino acids also control blood clotting in and around the placenta, keeping her safe. Protein molecules literally build your baby. Her brain development is highest in the third trimester, and your protein intake supports this developmental process.

For you

Protein gives your body the power to keep up with the demands of growing a baby.

It fills you up and keeps you satisfied for longer, helping to reduce cravings for chocolates and sweets, because it stabilizes blood sugar.

A protein-deficient diet can make mothers feel weak and light headed, have lowered immune systems and retain more fluid. Protein deficiency can also cause blood pressure to increase; protein is a blood pressure stabilizer.

How much do we need?

The general guideline of pregnancy is 90 grams as the daily target for protein. However, the 'one size fits' all approach doesn't resonate well with me as there are too many lifestyle factors to consider: type and frequency of exercise, weight, body mass index, and level of stress all play a role in how much you need. Having said that, we do need more than we think and a good guide would be between 70-90 grams daily.

Ask yourself 'where is my protein?' when you look down at each plate and snack you have throughout the day. Making a conscious effort to include protein with every meal and snack will help to ensure you are getting enough.

Sources of protein

Animal sources
Most people think meat when they think protein. I often am told, "Yes, I have protein: I eat chicken/fish once a day." That's great, but it's important to consider and include vegetable sources as well. If you are a meat eater, ideally you will be sourcing organic, grass-fed or pasture-raised meat sources.

Eggs are a great protein source and a pregnancy super food. A medium-sized egg has about 7 grams of protein. Make sure to buy free range!

Vegetarian sources
Being a vegetarian I love talking about plant-based protein. Years of living in India and counselling vegetarians and vegans taught me a lot about vegetarian protein sources and that it is possible to have a very

healthy pregnancy without meat. It does take a little more planning to get your daily requirement, but it is very do-able!

Good vegetarian protein sources include:

- Beans: kidney beans, navy beans, black beans, chickpeas, sprouted grains

- Lentils: black, brown, red, yellow

- Grains: amaranth, bulgur, quinoa, oats, sprouted grains

- Nuts: cashews, almonds, pistachio, walnuts, hazelnuts, Brazil nuts

- Seeds: pumpkin, hemp, chia, sunflower, sesame, flax

- Greens: kale, spinach, broccoli, asparagus

Whether you are a vegetarian or not, it is important to include these different plant-based sources, because they have a variety of healthy amino acids your body needs.

Personally, I do not recommend soy products like tofu because of their estrogen content and because many of them are genetically modified. Soy can confuse your thyroid and your body's own production of estrogen.

Please don't drink soymilk, especially during pregnancy. If you love soy products ensure they are organic, not genetically modified, and limit yourself to one or two servings a week.

Other protein sources to avoid during pregnancy include:

- Unpasteurized milk and cheese

- Raw fish

- Fish with high levels of mercury (swordfish)

- Processed meats (deli meats)

Quick ways to add protein

- Start the day with protein, whether from eggs, a green smoothie, oats, or peanut butter on toast.

- Prepare a seed mix, store it in a glass jar, and sprinkle it on your salads and soups.

- Choose peanut butter instead of jam for your toast.

- Make a batch of hummus at the start of the week to have in the fridge for snacking.

- Keep nuts like brazil, walnut, cashews in your purse for snacks.

There are lots of easy ways to incorporate more protein into your day.

"One of the most endearing things he (my partner) did during pregnancy was to look after my nutrition – always feeding me green juices and making sure I had enough food intake. He really was amazing support."
Amber, first baby, USA/Singapore

Probiotics and microbiome

Building a healthy microbiome is the latest thing sweeping the health world. Ensuring healthy gut flora is important during pregnancy, because you will also be "seeding" your baby's healthy flora at birth as she passes through the vagina and as you breastfeed. It will also help you to avoid candida outbreaks and keep your immune system strong.

Ways to increase your healthy gut and vaginal flora include eating fermented foods such as kombucha, kefir, fermented vegetables, pickles, and sauerkraut; taking daily probiotics.

Healthy fats

Health fats are essential for healthy tissues, so I've covered them in a special section on healthy tissues in Chapter 13.

Do

- Remember you are setting up your baby's food preferences: keep your nutrition varied and include lots of fresh vegetable with a rainbow of colors.

- Google-search for the foods highest in vitamin C, calcium and iron, and add more of the ones you like to your daily diet.

- Start noticing how much daily protein you take in, increase as needed.

- Learn all about healthy fats.

- Do some research on microbiome to learn more.

- Evaluate your food intake and decide whether you need supplements. Consider adding someone to your team who can help you.

SECTION 2

Opening

CHAPTER 11

....

What Does Your Baby Want?

"We must behave with the most enormous respect toward this instant of birth, this fragile moment. The baby is between two worlds. On a threshold. Hesitating. Do not hurry. Do not press. Allow this child to enter."

Fredrick Leboyer, obstetrician and author

The importance of making the shift from fear to love during pregnancy as we prepare for birth is as much for our baby's sake as it is for ourselves. We want to consider their experience as well as our own.

The American Academy of Pediatrics came out with the following statement in 2016: "Newborns are experiencing too much pain during routine medical procedures. Research suggests that repeated exposure to pain early in life can create changes in brain development and the body's stress response systems that can last into childhood."[3.]

The baby's experience

Babies are active participants in the process of birth; when we make decisions, both as PCPs and as parents, we need to consider the baby's experience too. There are two different scenarios of labor from the

....

[3.] "Early repetitive pain in preterm infants in relation to the developing brain", Manon Ranger and Ruth E Grunau
https://www.ncbi.nlm.nih.gov/pmc/articles/PMC3975052/

baby's perspective to consider: one filled with love and one filled with fear. One is not wrong or the other right; they are simply imagined perspectives of labor and birth for the little ones we carry.

"It's too cramped in here, and I need more space. But how am I going to get out of here and into my mother's arms?" That's your baby's first big problem to solve. Somewhere around 40 weeks old, baby is warm and safe, and yet needs to cross a bridge into the unknown. Maybe she remembers at some level the previous leap of faith and how well that went – specifically, that several day-old embryo leaping from the cozy Fallopian tube into a vast, black space, trusting it would land in the womb. There is an instinctive confidence mixed with excited anticipation, and baby begins storing up resources.

An epic journey filled with fear

Mother is screaming, breathing shallowly and completely tense with fear; her body is awash with stress hormones. Her care provider won't let her get off the bed or off her back, which feels like it is breaking. She hasn't been allowed to eat for eight hours; she feels like she is slowly dying.

Baby is quiet, feeling panicked; "what is happening to Mother? What is happening to me? These squeezes started out OK, but now everything is so tight and constricted." He keeps getting pushed down onto something hard and tight. His head is starting to hurt. He wishes Mother would relax; he wishes Mother would breathe.

Mother is done. She can't do this lying on her back. She wishes the nurses would just let her get up and walk to the bathroom to empty her bladder. She knows if she could move, she would be able to work with this intensity. But she cannot, and everyone is telling her about the dangers of getting up: "What if the cord falls down?"

She didn't want it, but she can't go on like this; it is time for an epidural. It feels like an eternity, but the anesthetist finally turns up, and the catheter and drugs are put into her spine. She relaxes.

Baby notices the relief of some additional space. Mother is breathing more quietly; things are softening. We can do this! He resumes moving his head from side to side, slowing burrowing in her direction; he smiles.

But now what's happening? Everything is fuzzy; a strange tingling sensation comes over his body. He is feeling sleepy and cannot keep his eyes open. So sleepy! "How do I get out of here and sleep at the same time?" Voices become muffled, and the baby drifts off to sleep.

Sometime later, he is jolted awake, and this water world has become fierce. The squeezes are intense, coming quickly one after another. Through the fog and grog, baby remembers what the mission was and starts again, pushing his head downwards, but there is no time, no rest. The bones are not moving. There is no space and everything is too tight. He can't get into the right position. He starts to feel panicked, "How will I get out of here? Why do I feel so weird? Why is the hugging so strong and fast? Is Mother OK? Where did she go?"

Baby woke up because Mother received a Pitocin drip after the surges slowed down following the epidural. She is sleeping comfortably on her back; Dad is also resting on the couch, and the nurses are busy in another room. No one notices that the drip is on too fast, and the mechanically produced surges are now too strong – titanic even. Baby is stressed, panicked. Signs of the distress start to show on the monitor as baby's heart rate accelerates and then decelerates.

Baby wants to thrash around to get someone's attention, but is too tired, too numb to do so. He whispers, "Mother, please help." And through the magic that they share, she stirs and looks at the monitor, then panics and rings the bell for the nurse.

This is a story you have probably heard many times before: fetal distress is discovered and an emergency Caesarean is called. The last line of the story is always the same: "Thank goodness for medical advances. Thank goodness we were in a hospital. Thank goodness the doctor came in to save the day. That was too close!"

What no one acknowledges, however, is that it is possible that the protocols of the advanced system put the baby at risk in the first place.

Consider the alternative scenario.

An epic journey filled with love and connection

Mother is moaning and swaying; her arms are around the neck of a person she loves. The room is dim, and the music she likes is playing. She feels relaxed and supported; her body is oozing oxytocin and endorphins. Someone says something funny and she laughs. She is so relieved that *today* is finally here, her birthing day. She feels ready.

Baby is feeling determined; he feels like he is working as part of a bigger team. The tight hugs from the uterine walls are manageable because mother is breathing and relaxing. There isn't much space, but there is enough. "Keep moving," he whispers to Mother with his mind, because he knows it is helping him find the way through the maze. The hugs are helping him. They push him downwards toward the exit. He can feel the subtle give that is happening: millimeter by millimeter something is changing, the way is opening.

> "A roller coaster ride! But we worked hard as a team, and the longer I labored, the more in tune I felt with my baby and recognized his immense role in birthing himself at the rate and pace he needed. When he was born, he was so calm, peaceful and alert. I did everything to protect the sanctity of our birth process because I wanted that to be his first gift: freedom to come gently, to be welcomed in a respectful way and to be celebrated as an equal birthing partner."
> Stacey Lee, first baby, South Africa/Singapore (breech birth)

Mother is moaning louder. With the sound she is making, her voice is calling him out. Everything softens again, and the feeling changes on his head as he feels himself slip an inch forward. "We can do this!" Then there is the sound of water running, "Our bath time! I love those! Is that what happens next? This is incredible! I am so strong; I am getting to Mother!"

And inch by inch he pushes forward and out; it is scary: he doesn't know how much further or longer the path is, but he feels Mother helping. And then something touches his head, he feels space, and water and movement. He is being lifted and then sound becomes louder, "Is this where I was going," he wonders? "Where is Mother?"

> "My baby would say Mum was in this with him 100%. We didn't give up, talked it out, and pushed one another until we met on the other side…and when we did, it was love at first sight!"
> Tanishq, first baby, India/Singapore

"I hear her, I feel her, I am still with her, now on top of her heart instead of under. Let me call out to her."

And he inflates his lungs and lets out a cry or perhaps simply inflates his lungs and has a look around.

Birth is one of the major events in life that imprints itself our nervous systems. We will not all have the gentle birth that we imagine for our babies, and that is OK, too. However, we should set it up to be as gentle as it can be, keeping their experience in the foreground. You might consider including in the team you are building people who can help if birth doesn't go as you plan.

Finding the food source

The second problem-solving opportunity for the baby at birth is how to get to the food source.

The more old-fashioned way of getting baby to the breast was by physically helping the baby – a nurse or midwife with one hand on baby's head and one hand on the mother's breast manually bringing them together.

Today, however, we favor allowing the baby time and space to find the breast herself. This search for food opens more new learning pathways in the brain and helps the baby feel confident. The mother also benefits: she is amazed how smart her little one is and feels a rush of confidence in their collective abilities.

This exploration is known as 'breast crawl', and is a beautiful process to witness. Nature thinks of everything, down to the smallest details, and has created absolute perfection. Have you ever wonder why your nipples get darker during pregnancy? For the baby's benefit! Babies see shades rather than colors at birth, and those darkened areolas are acting as a flashing target: "I'm over here! Come and get me!"

The process goes something like this: Around ten minutes old, instinct takes over, baby is on a mission again. Little arms stretch out in search for the nipple, then return to the mouth to see what has been found. All baby's senses have been heightened by the birth process, and to make up for their shallow field of vision (6-12 inches). Some babies lead by taste, and this stretching of arms and returning them to the mouth happens repeatedly, until there is a clear smell trail to follow from mouth to breast colostrum. Others lead by smell: they get a whiff of the sweet glory and start moving in that direction, one head bob and one kick at a time.

Baby coming straight up and onto his mother's bare chest provides another advantage: the familiar smell of amniotic fluid is on her chest, which also helps him to relax and feel safe in this new environment.

It is safe to assume that all babies have a headache after the birth; they used their heads to burrow through a pretty tight pathway. What the baby wants to soothe this headache is to suckle at the breast as soon as possible. It is like taking a Paracetamol. Remember, Mother has been high on endorphins and oxytocin during the birth process, and these hormones are in the colostrum.

If the baby is separated from the mother because of an immediate concern, she can still get all these benefits. They will just have to happen later and could be more challenging because he will likely have a nervous system slightly more on overdrive by that point.

> **Note:** if the baby is not finding her way to the breast, then of course we can help! There are no hard and fast rules here – only a suggestion to allow the time and space for the baby to find it herself to begin with.

Microbiome

A baby also needs the precious gift of healthy bacteria – a healthy microbiome. It's all about bugs.

We are living organisms, covered in and crawling with healthy "bugs": our microbes. The more microbes we have, the healthier we are, the stronger our immune systems are, and the less chance we have of developing allergies, asthma, eczema, and more.

Interestingly, the best time to get a strong, lifelong jump start with these healthy bugs is at birth, and that is why nature decided babies need to be born from 'down there' – Yup, next to the anus and going through all those vaginal juices. Coming in contact with the flora is what switches on and begins to build your baby's immune system.

To ensure we have good, healthy vaginal flora – filled with as many good bugs as possible – during pregnancy, we can do the following:

- take probiotics;
- eat fermented foods like kefir/kombucha/sauerkraut;

- take vitamin C and other immune support, and have Epsom salt baths;

- reduce stress and lightening our workloads;

- increase our self-love, making it a habit to relax and breathe every day, and enjoy exercise, yoga, and guided meditations; and

- avoid antibiotics

To make sure that the birth itself offers your baby the greatest exposure to good bugs, you'll need to

- prevent the hospital staff from wiping off the baby's vernix (the white cream on the baby's skin);

- delay the baby's first bath – I recommend not giving the first submersion bath until after the cord falls off, roughly 5-10 days after birth;

- avoid using soap, shampoo, creams or powders on the baby's skin; the only product I recommend using until six months old is coconut oil;

- give your baby immediate skin-to-skin contact and breastfeeding: they pick up lots of awesome microbes while rooting around on your chest to find the nipple;

- avoid antibiotics during labor; and

- put away hand sanitizers; simple soap and water after changing diapers and when interacting with baby will do.

On LoveBasedbirth.com you will find more information on the microbiome, with a great five-minute animation video. There is also a feature-length film, *Microbirth*, which you can watch it online for free – there are more details in the resources section at the back of the book.

·······
Do
·······

- Visualize your birth again, this time from the baby's perspective. What are the overriding emotions and feelings that you want your baby to experience?

- Learn more about microbiome.

- Watch the breast crawl video on LoveBasedBirth.com

Think about what your baby would like to see included on your birth plan:

- a PCP who will respect your birth preferences for a gentle birth;

- for you to breathe and relax as much as possible during labor and birth;

- for you to stay in communication with her during the birth process; she is scared too. (Regardless what type of birth you are having – home water birth, hospital birth with an epidural, or on the operating table – your baby wants to feel you connected to the process and to your breath.)

- for you to use as few drugs as possible during pregnancy and birth;

- for you to be upright and mobile as much as possible during labor, to help him find his way out (if you have an epidural ask your birth partner to help you move from side to side frequently);

- to come straight to you after birth, to be given time to land, relax, and hear your voice above all other sounds;

- to receive all his blood after birth – no early cord clamping;

- to be given time to find his food;

- to get all the healthy microbes, and not be bathed for at least the first few days;

- tons of skin-to-skin contact;

- no baby gloves; she wants to feel her environment to help her become confident;

- no perfumes and chemicals on her clothes (natural laundry soap recipe available on LoveBasedBirth website);

- not to get passed around to too many visitors to begin with;

- not to go to the nursery;

- not to be left alone with an unfamiliar paediatrician or other hospital staff.

CHAPTER 12

....

Birth Interventions

*"The woman in labor must have no stress placed upon her. She must
be free to move about, walk, rock, go to the bathroom by herself,
lie on her side or back, squat or kneel, or anything she finds
comfortable, without fear of being scolded or embarrassed.
Nor is there any need for her to be either 'quiet' or 'good.'
What is a 'good' patient? One who does whatever she
is told-who masks all the stresses she is feeling?
Why can she not cry, or laugh, or complain?"*
Grantly Dick-Read MD, obstetrician

The number of routine interventions used during birth is increasing.
Therefore, as healthy mums wanting a gentle birth for our babies, we
need a good understanding of what is necessary and what is not. We
will explore some of the main interventions in this chapter.

When a new mum walks into my office for a biodynamic craniosacral
session for herself and the baby, I start where I always do: "Tell me
about your pregnancy." I want to know things like: was it planned?
How did you feel being pregnant? Did you feel a connection with your
baby? And the next question is always: "Tell me about your birth."

Often, she is in my office because her little one has been given a
'problem child' label by a family member, another professional in the
community, or from her own diagnosis. It is a label that is often based
on the baby being hard to settle, 'fighting' the breast while feeding,

and having frequent bouts of uncontrollable crying or troubles with digestion.

I hear many variations of this story.

"I feel lucky to have had a normal birth, but unfortunately, I vomited for a large portion of the labor because of the side effects of the epidural. Then I needed a vacuum to help the baby out, because I was too tired."

Epidurals and vacuums can be necessary, but when did we start referring to them as normal or natural? We need the facts and a definition of normal.

- A baby born out of the vagina, with medications or any pharmaceutical support or any force other than the mother's, is a vaginal birth.

- A baby born without medications or pharmaceutical support of any kind, and with only the force from the mother, is a normal or natural birth.

Stay with me here: there is some debate about the use of the words "normal" and "natural". Considering birth is normal, how can normal be anything other than natural? Why, then, are we making a distinction between normal births and natural births? How did we get to the point where births that use interventions are called normal? Got it?

> **Disclaimer:** once again – I am not anti-intervention and I am grateful that all the interventions exist, because they can be lifesaving. However, I question their overuse and popularity.

Here is a list of common interventions:

- Induction/augmentation
- Breaking the water bag

- Pain medication: epidural, pethidine, gas and air, etc.
- Intravenous (IV) drips
- Episiotomy
- Vacuum/forceps
- Fundal pressure
- Caesarean
- Enema
- Hospital gowns
- Restricting fluids/food
- Antibiotics
- Monitoring straps
- Continuous monitoring
- Urine catheter
- Constant fetal monitoring
- Stirrups
- Lying flat in bed to give birth
- Vaginal examinations
- Any position that is not your choice
- Anyone observing the birth not invited by the mother
- Suctioning a healthy newborn
- Immediate cord clamping/cutting
- Separating the newborn from the mother

Even observing and making suggestions can be considered interventions. The best doulas and midwives sit quietly in the corner, not interfering unless the mother requests.

Interventions typically snowball or cascade, one into another. For example, if you get an epidural, you will also automatically get:

- An IV drip
- A urine catheter
- Monitoring straps
- Restricted food/fluids

… and you will have a higher chance of also getting:

- Pitocin
- Vacuum/forceps
- Fundal pressure (exerting pressure on the abdomen to hasten the second stage of labor)
- Separation from baby immediately after the birth
- Caesarean

Seven common interventions

Here we will look at seven of the interventions routinely on offer in hospitals. (More information on common labor interventions can be found on LoveBasedbirth.com.)

1. Induction/Augmentation

The difference between induction and augmentation is that induction is what is done to get labor started in the first place, and augmentation is what is used to speed it up once it is already in process. Many women are taken down this path unnecessarily, based on the PCP's lack of experience, expertise or patience.

Induction is the number one intervention you want to avoid if you are planning a normal birth. Once you start tricking the body with synthetic hormones, your own essential birth hormones like oxytocin and endorphins are not going to work in the same way. That is why induction tends to be matched with an epidural: if your body is no longer creating its own sensations, they will be very different, with surges often coming too fast, making them too much and too hard to manage.

This doesn't mean that if you require an induction, you need to throw out your birth preferences and take whatever is coming. No – go one step at a time, and let your body know you have given the drugs permission to be there, and that your body can accept them with ease because they are needed.

When interviewing your PCP, ask early on what their most common reasons for induction are. If any of these reasons are on the list, you know you are not with an evidenced-based care provider. None of these reasons on their own are medical indications for induction:

- Cord around the neck
- Baby too big
- Past 40 weeks
- IVF conception

On the subject of cords, I hear this all too often: *"I was induced/given a Caesarean/had a vacuum delivery because my baby's cord was around his neck."* This is a *huge* myth in medical models of birth. In fact, 50% of babies are born with the cord around their necks. It is normal, totally natural.

Can it cause problems? Yes of course. Anything is possible during birth, just as it is possible to be hit by a car when you cross the street or to trip on something you didn't see coming and break your knee. But are these reasons to not leave the house or to not walk? Or reasons to be proactive and pay attention to where we are going?

From another perspective, you could ask whether around the neck is the safest place for the cord to be, because it keeps it out of the way of the head as it burrows its way out.

2. Restricting food and drink

Imagine running a marathon without being able to have nourishment along the way. There would be more leg cramps, many more drop-outs and probably more ambulances called. Labor is no different: you need to be able to keep your energy levels up. The uterus is a muscle, and it needs fuel to work at its best. Many hospitals are still following the practice of starving women during labor, when research shows:

> "Most healthy women can skip the fasting and, in fact, would benefit from eating a light meal during labor. The research suggests that the energy and caloric demands of laboring women are similar to those of marathon runners."
> The American Society of Anesthesiologists

3. Constant fetal monitoring

Research shows that if you and your baby are healthy and do not have any risk factors like heart disease, diabetes or high blood pressure, and you are not on an epidural or any other drugs during labor, constant monitoring of the fetal heart rate does not improve outcomes. What it does increase is the likelihood of a Caesarean delivery.[4] Constant monitoring means being strapped into a bed, and being in a bed will greatly decrease your chances of a normal birth. Why? Because laboring in a bed is far from normal.

....
[4] Alfirevic, Z., D. Devane, et al. (2006). "Continuous cardiotocography (CTG) as a form of electronic fetal monitoring (EFM) for fetal assessment during labour." Cochrane database of systematic reviews(3): CD006066.

At the birth center in Kerala, our first birth on the bed only happened in our second year. The bed is a huge king-size, but women could birth where they pleased. They had options: a water birth pool, a hanging rope, a birth stool, and floor space. The point is, instinct would never prompt you to get on a bed and lie on your back to have a baby. That is something invented by a man, by an institution for their convenience.

4. Antibiotics

Overuse of antibiotics is making our world's population sick, and antibiotic-resistant strains of bacteria are on the rise. We have discussed throughout this book the importance of protecting and boosting your microbiome, as well as building a healthy microbiome for your baby during pregnancy. If you have routine antibiotics during labor, in part, your hard work is wasted.

There are some situations when antibiotics may be necessary; discuss them with your care provider. Research shows that using antibiotics in labor for the following reasons can indeed have a benefit for mums and babies:

- Waters open longer than 24 hours
- Fever during labor
- Prematurity

The reasons for giving should *not* include

- "We administer them routinely"
- "Just in case your waters open"
- "Because you have Group B streptococcus and your waters might break"

5. Flat on your back/in stirrups

Remember we are human mammals. Have you ever seen a goat, a horse or an elephant lie down and put their legs in the air to give birth? It doesn't happen.

Forward-leaning positions take the pressure off your back and provide access for someone to give you counter-pressure or massage your back. They support your pelvis and sacrum to open as it needs to; lying on your back reduces your pelvic dimensions, and allow for coping better with the birth sensations. You are not meant to labor in a bed. Birthing flat on your back will also increase your risk of perineal damage (all of the pressure of the baby's head is on it.)

It is also curious that women are warned to not lie or sleep on their backs in pregnancy because it might restrict blood flow, but it is perfectly OK for them to spend eight+ hours of labor in that position That doesn't make sense at the time when the chance of blood flow interruption is at its highest.

6. Intravenous drips

In many hospitals, the routine practice includes having an IV drip in your arm for hydration. Some would see this as a benign intervention. Does it matter if I have a drip?

Yes, it does. If you have routine IV fluids during labor, it means being attached to an IV pole, so your movement will be restricted. It will also have the effect of making you feel subconsciously sick and weak, instead of feeling, 'the most powerful you have ever been'. It can cause trouble with breastfeeding as receiving and retaining too much fluid can cause more engorgement of the breast tissue and increased pain. Routine IV use in labor has been linked with babies with excessive weight loss. In fact, they have not done so, but their weight was artificially higher at birth because they had retained fluid and become puffy from the hours of IV fluid.

Some hospitals use drips as reasons to restrict your oral fluid intake: "You have the drip, so you don't need to worry about drinking."

Like everything, there are instances where you may need an IV, for example, if you have been vomiting and are dehydrated, or if you are exhausted and need more energy.

7. Hospital gowns

I was in the role of a doula with a woman who was having a planned hospital birth for her third baby. We arrived at the hospital in rock and roll labor, and the nurse came in and handed her a gown, "Here, put this on."

Without missing a beat, after a strong surge that brought her forward to rest her weight on her arms on the side of the bed, she turned round to the nurse and said, "For all I know, someone died in that gown yesterday and if you think I am going to wear it today, think again."

My jaw dropped in surprise, as did the nurse's.

Birth is a mental process. Hospital gowns have an aura of sickness and weakness, just like a wheelchair – say no to that, too, and walk up to the labor and delivery suite.

Making decisions

A question that comes up frequently is: "When will I know if I *truly* need the intervention being suggested by my PCP?" It will be easier if you have chosen a PCP who your intuition has guided you to trust. Building a relationship of trust prenatally is key to feeling confident with whatever is being suggested during labor.

Decisions aren't always black and white. Being an informed consumer is important, but don't feel you have to complete a PhD on labor and birth during pregnancy.

"We had several twists and turns from our planned birth. (Changing from home to hospital birth) a breech presentation and waters opening 70+ hours before baby arrived. My husband and I just stayed focused on making decisions that aligned with our philosophy and outlook on life. We remained calm and trusted that my body and baby were doing exactly what they needed to do. Also we knew that we had choices. And that the choices were for us to make and not to be forced to choose something that we didn't want."

Amanda, first (breech) baby, USA/Singapore

BRAIN is a simple way to help you make an informed decision in the moment:

B – What are the benefits?

R – What are the risks?

A – What are the alternatives?

I – What is my intuition saying?

N – What if we do nothing?

Remember you *always* have options.

"There were a lot of twists and turns (during my birth) the opening took very long, I needed an epidural after 36 hours and after 45 hours hormones (Pitocin) to help the opening. I stayed calm, discussed with my husband and we made the decisions together. The team was great, they never pushed us in a decision and we were confirmed that we can fully trust them. It really showed the importance of choosing a provider you can fully trust to respect your wishes."

Anonymous, second baby, Singapore

....
Do
....

- Be clear about what interventions are routine in your place of birth and with your PCP.

- Plan to avoid all the small interventions to avoid the bigger ones.

- Consider the common routine interventions when putting together your birth preferences.

- Enroll in a birth preparation class taught by an independent educator. You want someone who will teach you how to have an informed birth, not how to be a good patient.

- Go to LoveBasedBirth.com to find templates and step-by-step information to create your birth preferences/plan.

CHAPTER 13

·····················

Stretching And Preparing To Open

I have never observed even the slightest laceration in a woman who used clitoral stimulation as a relaxation method during birth. Clitoral stimulation seems to increase vaginal engorgement as the baby emerges.

Ina May Gaskin, midwife, author

"How on earth is my body going to open and stretch to the degree required to give birth? My vagina is quite small." I hear that a lot. You might be sitting there wondering the same thing right now. You might have been asking yourself a similar question at the beginning of your pregnancy. "How will my body stretch to fit an entire person inside?"

Thankfully, stretching is a gradual process; we don't wake up one morning with a basketball-sized baby in our bellies. Step by step and inch by inch, our body expands to accommodate the person growing inside us. Our organs move to the side and our stomach muscles separate, to allow the space the baby needs.

The constant comments from strangers don't help – we are surely too big or too small. As there is a 50% chance of being deemed 'too big', our fear could keep growing along with our bellies. I find it sad that we live in a world where we don't all make an effort to be kind and encouraging when we see pregnant women.

As I am less than 5 feet tall, my baby didn't have anywhere to go but straight out early on in pregnancy. By the time I was 20 weeks, I was always being asked if I was having twins or if I was sure my baby wasn't due until May. I kept looking down, thinking, what is going to happen to this belly in another 20 weeks if it is already this big? Then somewhere around 24 weeks, I was in a restaurant and an older woman behind the counter beamed at me, "You look beautiful!" I don't mind admitting that comment bounced joyfully around in my head all day. When you feel worried about your expanding body and the stretch needed for birth, just think of all the babies that have grown and been born since the beginning of time, and of their mothers, who probably had similar concerns.

UNICEF estimates that around 353,000 babies are born each day around the world; that is 255 births globally per minute or 4.3 births every second (December 2013 estimate). That is a lot of women stretching beautifully, many of them with twins and triplets.

Growing a human is a big deal both mentally and physically, and it is one of the greatest opportunities to trust in the magic and mystery of the unimaginable.

There are three things that make expanding and stretching easier. Let's look at them in the context of both pregnancy and birth:

- Lubrication

- Relaxation

- Healthy tissues

Lubrication

During birth, your vagina will naturally be lubricated with birth juices. Your amniotic water may be leaking with each surge. Your mucus plug might be coming out bit by bit, or you might have some blood spotting as your baby's head nudges your cervix open. You might even have the moist cushion of the amniotic sac still surrounding the baby's head, if your waters haven't opened. Some babies are actually born inside their amniotic sacs.

The lubrication of our tissue and skin during pregnancy is related to how hydrated we keep ourselves. Doing your best to stay hydrated: about 3 liters of water a day, depending on the climate you live in and how much you sweat, is ideal. For many women, it is difficult to drink water during the first trimester, and that is OK. Don't pressure yourself; go with the flow in the first trimester. It will probably feel good to get back to drinking water once the second trimester starts.

I am a big fan of drinking coconut water to keep the body hydrated. It is a perfect blend of electrolytes and is similar to blood plasma. In World War II, some patients were given coconut water as an intravenous solution when saline wasn't available. If you are following Chinese medicine, coconut is not recommended in the first trimester, because of its cooling effect on the body, but it can be drunk in the second and third trimesters.

Lubrication of the skin is also important during pregnancy. Using coconut oil to massage your belly and breasts daily is a good practice to start in the first trimester. If you live in a cold climate, you might want to use a more warming oil, like olive or almond. I have a very old Indian Ayurvedic pregnancy book, and it advises that avoiding stretch marks on the breasts during pregnancy requires a daily 5-minute massage of the breasts with coconut oil for the duration of the first trimester. It worked for me!

Some midwives pour olive oil or coconut oil on the perineum during birth, while the baby is crowning, to help the tissues to stretch. I haven't used this method, because I haven't seen the need, but it is a point you could discuss with your PCP if the idea appeals to you.

Relaxation

It is common to hear about the benefits of doing pelvic floor exercises to strengthen the pelvic floor during pregnancy, but we don't hear much about learning to soften and relax it, which is equally important. Whether we know it or not, we can hold a lot of tension in our perineum (the area between the vagina and the anus). You may be clenching that area without being aware of it, especially when you are fearful, stressed or overwhelmed with busyness. I invite you to spend time actively being aware of your perineum throughout the day and noticing when it is tense and when it is relaxed.

We were taught from an early age to tense up in order to let go (think of having a poo). However, the body doesn't like that. As a result, constipation, piles and hemorrhoids are quite common for many people, caused not only by poor diet, but also poor elimination habits.

It is the same at birth. We all have an image in our minds of the red-faced woman in the movie, holding her breath, clenching her jaw and facial muscles as someone shouts, "*Push!*" and counts down from ten. Blood vessels are popping in her face as she strains and clenches.

That is not the way to give birth to a baby gently.

To let anything go out of our bodies, it makes sense to soften and breathe into the sensation rather than brace against it. It still requires effort, but one that is more softened and internally focused. The best place to practice this theory is on the toilet.

Next time you have the urge to poo try this: sit on the toilet, relax, and find your breath. Focus on your anal sphincter and perineum, and see if you can relax it so much that it feels like it bulges gently outward. Find your breath and breathe into your diaphragm. As you exhale, relax your whole bottom area even further, and imagine your breath traveling down and filling that area. Feel how you can gently, internally nudge your breath down. With practice, gas will start to move, and then your bowel will empty. This practice has helped many people – men and women– that I have worked with to overcome elimination issues.

Ideally, this is what you will do while moving your baby down at the time of birth, as well: soften into the feeling, rather than tightening and bracing against it. I can see that the more relaxed a mum is while her baby is emerging, the less tearing she has. When she has a smile on her face, the baby seems to slide out so much more easily, and tears rarely occur. This is the mirror principle we talked about in Chapter 10: soft, open lips and jaw = soft, open vulva and vagina.

> **CASE STUDY**
>
> I was talking to a new mum from my birth preparation class who came in for a BCST session with her baby. She was telling me how she ended up with far more intervention than she planned: the baby was posterior positioned, so she opted for an epidural and the help of a vacuum to birth him.
>
> He weighed 4400g, but even with all that intervention, she didn't need any stitches. She said that during the time she was working to move the baby all the way down until he was out, she was consciously softening her jaw, her lips – doing everything we had practiced together. I was so proud of her: it just goes to show that birth can sometimes unfold differently from how we imagined, but if it does, all the things you spent time learning beforehand will still benefit you a lot.

Midwives are well known for their abilities to gently encourage mums and to "whisper" babies out. You want to be sure your PCP is well versed in supporting babies to be born gently, and ideally *between* surges.

I love this passage in Fredrick Leboyer's book, *Birth Without Violence*, first published in 1974:

> "This apprenticeship of silence – so indispensable for mothers – is just as important for those who perform the delivery: the obstetricians, the attendants.
>
> People speak loudly in the delivery room. The calls to 'push, push' are rarely whispered. So profoundly wrong.

These loud outbursts upset the mother more than help her.

Lowered voices can relax her, and do far more for her than shouting.

Those who assist in deliveries must learn this new silence. They too must be prepared to receive the child with care and respect."

Perineal massage

I believe in the wisdom of the body too much to buy into the idea that you need to stretch your vaginal tissues hundreds of times before birth for them to stretch with ease over the baby's head. Having said that, I do see that perineal massage has a role to play, and this is why:

1. Massaging is more for your mind than your tissues. Birth is as much a mental as it is a physical exercise. Perineal massage during pregnancy may enable you to become more connected with your body and to reduce fears about birth. Becoming familiar with the sensation of stretching prenatally could help you to be more relaxed with the sensation of stretching at the time of birth. And softening into that relaxation is the ideal.

> **Note:** Some evidence has shown that massaging the perineum at the time of birth causes the tissues to become more edemous (filled with fluid), which makes them more susceptible to tearing. Therefore, find out what your PCP's policy on perineal massage during birth is.

2. Confidence is the key in this entire process, and however you build it up, go for it! You will never stretch the vaginal/perineal tissue yourself as much as your baby will, but you will at least get the feeling of it, so you have will have some idea of what to expect.

3. Do this with your partner. Perineal massage provides an opportunity to work together with a strong sensation while he/she helps you to relax and find your breath. Because of this, you will get more benefit doing it together than on your own.

You can find different ways to do perineal massage online, including on the Love Based Birth website.

Tips for perineal massage

Perineal massage is safe and does not interact with the cervix, so you don't have to wait until 36 weeks to give it a try.

- Use lots of lubrication I like coconut oil (are you seeing a theme here?), because it is both antifungal and antibacterial.

  - Incorporate it into your love-making, so the body is already soft and receptive. ("Hey babe, let's do a perineal massage", the minute you walk in the door from work, is not be what we are going for here!)

- Decide together before you start how far you want to go with the stretch, on a scale of 0 being nothing and 10 being the size of a baby's head. That will give you both an expectation to guide you. Your lover won't want to hurt you, and good communication will make you both feel more confident.

- Advice to the stretcher: make sure she is comfortable before you start. Put a towel under her bottom, and pour lots of oil on your hands and on her for lubrication. Insert your two thumbs or pointer fingers into her vagina, then pause and wait until she relaxes again. You can help her by directing her toward those belly breaths she has been practicing, inhaling into the ribs and down to the belly to for a count of three and exhaling for a count of six. Also, help her to relax any part of her body that she tightens – forehead, jaw, tummy muscles, butt muscles, fists, etc. Once she is relaxed, try a bit more of a stretch by giving gentle, but firm, upward and outward pressure at the base of the vaginal opening. Pause when she clenches, and help her relax again by finding her breath, and repeat.

There is a balloon that can do all this for you. If you haven't heard of the Epi-no, you might want to check it out. It is a balloon with a hand pump attached to it. The idea is that you insert it into the vagina, blow it up, to get used to the feeling of stretching. You can start slowly with a 4cm circumference, and gradually increase it until you get to 10 cm. I must admit I was slightly horrified when I first heard about it, but I now know many women who have used it, they swear by it. Seeing is believing, and I have seen the benefits for first-time mums who have used it prenatally. To date, none of them has had a tear that needed stitches. Bear in mind that using the Epi-no is not recommended until 36-37 weeks.

Healthy tissues

Another important factor that affects how your skin and tissues stretch during pregnancy and birth is the integrity, or elasticity, of your tissues. Two key ingredients for tissue elasticity are healthy fats and zinc:

Healthy fats include:

- Coconuts and coconut milk

- Flax seeds/flax oil

- Nuts: almonds, walnuts, cashews

- Avocados

- Dark chocolate

- Eggs

- Fatty fish

- Ghee

Make these foods part of your daily nutrition.

I like to say, "An avocado a day keeps the tear away." Avocados are widely available and very versatile. You can put one in your smoothie, make guacamole or pair it with just about every meal you can think of.

Zinc

The recommended daily dose during pregnancy is around 40 mgs. Taking folic acid, which you are advised to do during pregnancy, lowers the zinc levels in the body, so it is easy to see why it is possible to become zinc-depleted during pregnancy. Zinc deficiency has been associated with preterm labor, growth restriction, prolonged labor and more, all great reasons to include zinc in your diet.

Zinc-rich foods include:

- Cocoa powder
- Cashews
- Pumpkin seeds
- Yogurt/kefir
- Chickpeas
- Meats

> **Note:** Chose a natural supplement of Folate over Folic Acid. Folate is easier for the body to absorb. Please do your own research on folic acid verse folate, you might be surprised what you find.

If you get a tear...

The perineum is designed to tear at the time of birth, and it heals very well. The mucosa of the vagina is just like the mucosa of your mouth. Remember when you bit the inside of your cheek and it bled? Later that day you could probably feel with your tongue that a completely new layer had already formed. The vagina is the same, allowing high-speed cell regeneration for healing.

A natural tear heals much better than an episiotomy (when scissors are used to cut the tissues of the perineum to make the exit bigger for the baby) and has fewer long-term effects. The World Health Organisation has defined the episiotomy as an emergency procedure, which should only be used if the mother or baby is in danger, not routinely. Yet, sadly, it is still done by many PCPs around the globe.

Please discuss this issue with your doctor, and if you need more information about it, go to the Love Based Birth website and search for 'episiotomy'.

Read more about how you can prepare for healing after birth with sitz baths in Chapter 25.

Do

- Work on the three elements to support the stretch: lubrication, relaxation, and healthy tissues.

- Create a mental imagine that helps you to relax when you get anxious about stretching or anything else. (In the lead up to starting the stimulation process of IVF, I had a visual that I used all the time: I imagined a big comfy, purple velvet armchair – the type you could just melt into. Whenever I felt my anxiety rising, I would close my eyes and imagine settling back into that chair. It worked very well for me; I got into that chair a lot and always felt better.

- Remember your vagina is not a tube. If you think it is, then you might consider some further self-exploration. It is an incredible shape-shifter made up of many intricate folds designed to expand, open, receive, and gently hug whatever is there: a finger, penis, or a baby.

CHAPTER 14

....

Setting The Stage

"According to traditional wisdom in rural France, a baby in the womb should be compared to fruit on the tree. Not all the fruit on the same tree is ripe at the same time…we must accept that some babies need a much longer time than others before they are ready to be born."
Michel Odent MD, obstetrician, author

As we begin to build a visual picture of labor, ideally that picture will include gratitude: gratitude that labor is hard work. Gratitude that our cervix is so strong it can hold up an entire universe; gratitude that it will take hours of breathing and moving for the cervix to open and for baby to make its way down and into our arms.

Imagine the alternative: a weak cervix, one that opened easily? Babies would arrive at 25 weeks and 28 weeks and 32 weeks, in shopping malls and movie theatres, in the car and walking down the street!

We want to be better prepared for them than that. We want to be in a safe space, with people around us who we love, to help us celebrate and welcome them.

There is no way around it: labor is work, and this is a beautiful thing! In this chapter, we will have a general look at the beginning of opening up and expanding into another realm: the birth of a new human on the planet – and of a mother.

You might already have noticed that I use some birth terms that are different from what you commonly hear. Part of reclaiming birth as normal is using language that is positive and affirming, rather than dramatic and sometimes violent. We now have a better understanding of the power of language, the pictures and feelings it creates. This language is widely used among gentle birth educators. Here are some examples:

- "Surges" rather than "contractions" – not because contractions are painful and surges aren't, but because "surge" is a better description of what the uterine muscle is doing. Contractions means shortening when in fact the muscle is elongating. And when you watch a surge on a monitor, it looks exactly like a wave: it builds up to a peak, and then comes down the other side.

- Waters "opening/releasing" rather than waters "breaking/water rupturing": I'm not sure about you but the idea of something breaking or rupturing in my body is horrifying and sounds like an emergency.

Hormones in labor

There are three main hormones involved in the opening process: oxytocin, endorphins and relaxin.

Oxytocin is the love hormone. It is releases when we are having tea with a friend we like, looking at a beautiful sunset, and is highest when we are making love and having an orgasm. The job of oxytocin during labor is to create the surges. It is what causes the uterine muscle fibers to stretch up and back around the baby's head.

Essentially, the same hormone that got the baby in will get the baby out!

Oxytocin is also a shy hormone. It needs privacy and a feeling of safety to work at its best. Strangers and bright lights are not the ingredients oxytocin loves to work with. It is for oxytocin's sake that we want the environment we labor in to be non-threatening and calming, just like the environment we want to make love in.

Endorphins are the body's natural pain relievers, known to be 200 times stronger than morphine – how impressive is that? Also known as feel-good hormones, they are released when we do any physical activity, such as a vigorous workout, a yoga session, or a brisk walk; they are the reason why exercise is one of the antidotes to depression. During labor, endorphins are there to help you "get into the zone"; the longer and stronger you labor, the more endorphins are released and the easier it should be to flow with the rhythm of your body.

Relaxin softens all your ligaments, specifically those of your pelvis, creating more space for baby to maneuver through it. This hormone is present in the body at the start of pregnancy and builds towards birth. Relaxin is what causes that penguin walk at the end of the third trimester; your hips and pelvis might feel very wobbly.

While experiencing my own first pregnancy, women asked me all the time what surprised me most about it after so many years of working with pregnant women. Without a doubt, for me, it was relaxin! I was amazed at how early I felt my pelvis changing and opening, and how destabilizing that felt. How quickly I was unable to do any wide-legged yoga asanas without feeling like my ligaments were going to pull apart.

This is just another example of how different we all are. I was looking at some very impressive yoga photos on Instagram, photos of one of the women from my last birth preparation class. Her deep asanas made my wobbling pelvis sore just to look. My assumption was because she was already so flexible the effect of relaxin must be even more intense for her, but when I asked she replied, "Relaxin? No, I haven't noticed any difference in how my pelvis feels."

Oxytocin and endorphins are both secreted by the pituitary gland – an ancient part of the brain often associated with the brow chakra or clairvoyance in Eastern mysticism – and relaxin is secreted by the ovaries and the placenta. They are all part of your perfect design.

Birth timing

There is no such thing as an alarm bell that goes off at 40 weeks, or your "due date": all babies decide to be born at different times. The easiest way to calculate 40 weeks from your last period is to add a year and seven days then subtract three months.

A full-term pregnancy is considered as 37–42 weeks' gestation from your last period, assuming you have a 28- to 30-day cycle. If your cycle is longer or shorter, you will need to work with your PCP to adjust your expectations accordingly.

As discussed in Section 1, make sure your PCP is happy to monitor you and wait for you to go up to two weeks over the expected time without pressuring you, if you and the baby are happy and healthy.

The end of pregnancy is a mental game: your friends and family are probably messaging and asking you every day if anything is happening. They might have been doing that for weeks already. I encourage you to talk in terms of the month rather than the day. "My baby will be born sometime in May' was what I always said when asked. It can help to avoid the 'pressure pot' at the end of pregnancy. (You might even choose to give a date that is a few weeks later then the "estimated date of delivery".)

In the meantime, if you plan to go to hospital for birth, ensure your bag includes:

- Socks/slippers – hospital floors are cold

- Snacks –a mix of stuff as you don't know what you'll feel like at the time, but you want a variety of things to keep your energy up such as fruit, protein bars, honey bars

- Hydration drinks – coconut water is the best!

- A shawl or bathrobe – moving between feeling hot and cold is the norm, so having something easy to put on and off is great
- Your birth plan
- Speakers and headphones
- Battery candles or a string of white fairy lights

Natural ways to get things moving

If you are at 41 weeks and nothing is happening, these are some of the things you can do to encourage the body to begin letting go. Remember, if none of them works it is because the baby is simply not ready.

- Sex
- Acupuncture
- Acupressure
- Reflexology
- Belly massage
- Essential oils
- Homeopathy

Relax and breathe. Your baby is coming; up to 42 weeks is completely normal, for healthy mums and babies.

Stages of labor

The whole birth process is considered to be in three main parts:

1. First stage: labor
2. Second stage: fully dilated, the pushing part
3. Third stage: birth of the placenta

I break the first stage down further into four parts: early, active, rock and roll, and transformation. Each stage is basically an increased intensity from the one before. Women won't always know which one they are in, and the stages don't always correlate with how many centimeters of dilation the cervix has reached.

As a super generalization, we can say:

- Early labor = 0–3cm

- Active = 3–5cm

- Rock and roll = 6–8cm

- Transformation = 8–10cm

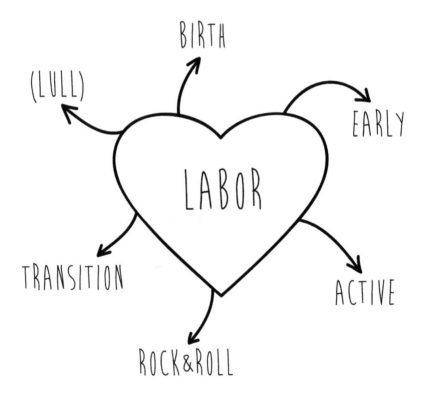

Remember, every birth is as different as each of us looks. To describe every potential variation of labor would have this book weighing 15kg in your hands right now. Keep in mind as we go through the stages that I am generalizing; you may not fit into any of this, and that wouldn't be surprising; however, the majority of first-time mums will.

Early labor

One of the key factors for how birth ends is how it is treated at the start. You would not start a marathon with a sprint, right? It's the same with birth: don't use up all your energy the starting line. The golden rule of labor is to rest and ignore it as long as possible. Early labor or warm-up labor is usually the longest part of the whole process, because it can start and stop for several days. You want to understand the difference between early and active labor to avoid getting to the hospital too early.

So how will you know you're in labor? From the surges – gentle, uterine hugs that will grow and build in intensity. If you are wondering if you are in labor, then you might still be days away from it. You will not mistake established labor, because there will be no question in your mind. All of your focus will be on your breath and on softening into the sensation.

To get an idea if we are in early or active labor, we can time the surges. When we do this, we are looking at both their duration and frequency. How often do they come, and how long do they last?

Early labor surges are usually irregular in both respects. If you were to plot them on a graph, they wouldn't make any clear pattern. The duration ranges from 10–45 seconds, and the frequency from 2–20 minutes apart. They are doing good preparation work – I don't believe in 'false' labor – but they are not yet opening you. They will probably be mild enough for you to talk while you are having one, continue with your activity (maybe slowing it down a bit), or think about something else while the gentle uterine hug is happening.

They are laying the labor groundwork by softening your cervix and moving it forward. The cervix is usually long and hard and feels a bit like a nose. It will need to become short and soft, feeling more like lips, before it will begin to open.

If irregular surges start at night:

- Stay in bed.

- Get into a cozy, side-lying position, with a pillow between your knees.

- Listen to your favorite relaxation track with your headphones.

- Take deep belly breaths.

- Sleep between the surges.

- Connect with your baby: tell her you are excited she is ready to make the move into your arms.

- Take sips of water.

If surges start during the day, have a distraction project. Try to find a balance between rest and activity. Here are some ideas:

- Keep a couple five-star movies you've been looking forward to seeing on standby.

- Bake a cake.

- Go for a nature walk.

- Take a bath.

- Do whatever else you like to do that keeps you engrossed.

Mostly you want to avoid looking at the clock or paying attention to every small sensation, wondering if *that one* is the real thing. Remember, this is a mental game. Don't exhaust yourself early.

What does a surge feel like? Every woman describes it differently:

- a tight hug
- a feeling of pressure
- a strong pulling sensation
- the most intense sensation I ever felt in my body
- strong menstrual cramps
- like my back was breaking
- pulling
- tightening
- stretching
- terrible pain

Your birth partner has an important role in early labor: to provide reassurance, distraction – and to possibly time some surges.

Do

- Remember the key to early labor is to ignore it and rest for as long as possible.
- Plan early labor projects for distraction, in case it starts during the day.

CHAPTER 15

Labor – The Bridge

"The parallels between making love and giving birth are clear not only in terms of passion and love, but also because we need essentially the same conditions for both experiences: privacy and safety."
Sarah J. Buckley MD

Now we are getting into the real work of labor. Up until now it has mostly been mental, but now we are turning the corner to include the physical.

Active labor

Active labor is the next longest part of the birth process after early labor. It is defined as the process of getting the cervix to open from 3 to 8cms, and the average timing can be anywhere from 4–8 hours. It might start with a bang or it might build slowly. The surges of active labor become more rhythmic. Each one is likely to last 60 seconds, and they will come at a frequency of every 4-6 minutes.

Surges for first-time mums need to last for 60 seconds before the cervix begins to open. As a rough guide – remember, we are all different – after an hour of a regular pattern of 60-second surges coming every 5 minutes, you are at the start of active labor. Once you are well established in these minute-long surges that are coming frequently and building in intensity, you won't be wondering if you are in labor anymore.

> "[I am proudest of] during pregnancy: the preparation, preparation, preparation we did. During labor: laboring at home for as long as possible, staying in the moment, adapting to my changing surroundings. During birth: gently birthing a breechling into the world, and in the face of many (potential) obstacles."
>
> Stacey Lee, first baby, breech birth, South Africa/Singapore

Is the start of active labor the time to go to your birthing location if it is not home? No. Ideally, you should spend most of your labor at home, especially if your planned location is a high-intervention hospital. A doula can help you to stay at home longer, and again there are things you can do in active labor to distract you from heading to the hospital:

- Take a bath or a warm shower.

- Stay in "conserve" mode for as long as possible – as long as you are comfortable relaxing on your side, in a chair, on hands and knees or in child's pose. (Do not feel like you *should* be moving, or walking; once it is time to move your body will tell you.)

- Every surge will stop you in your tracks to breathe and focus.

- Sway and circle your hips if that feels good.

- Stay connected with your baby – remember every surge is taking you one step closer to meeting her.

- Work to relax *with* the surge.

- Drink water between surges.

- Have a light snack.

- Empty your bladder every hour.

- Welcome the growing intensity; it is bringing your beautiful darling into your arms.

Birth partners: make sure she is staying hydrated and remind her to pee frequently. Pre-empt her needs and take care of all the details, so she only needs to be present with the surges.

Rock and roll labor

How do I know it is time to go to the hospital?

Rock and roll labor is when you will want to go to the hospital (assuming you live in a city and the hospital is 10–20 minutes away). I fondly refer to the later part of active labor as 'rock and roll' labor because it captures all your senses. It can't be ignored, and the more you let go into being carried by the music, the better the music will feel.

Once you enter rock and roll labor, you might naturally start vocalizing with sound breathing.

You will move slowly on your way to the car. It will take time to get to the door, time to get down in the lift, and time to get into the car/taxi. With each surge, you will pause, lean against the wall and breathe, spend a few seconds recovering, and then move on. If you can simply walk out the door and get into a car, it is too early! Go back inside, it is not time for the hospital yet – unless the hospital is several hours away.

I worked with a woman who spent a lot of time during pregnancy imagining herself as jelly, softening her entire body with her imaginary surges. She had spent so much time with that visualization practice that it was easy for her to re-enact it during labor. She told me with a smile after the birth, when I commented on how relaxed she was, "I just kept imagining I was softening my whole body into jelly. I couldn't fight it when I tried to be jelly instead."

That is what we control in labor: where our mind goes.

Transformation (also known as Transition)

Transformation is the most intense part of opening for most women. In an ideal world, you might be arriving at the hospital now or just settling in. When the labouring women is in charge rather than controlled or silenced, this is incredibly beautiful time of labor to witness. For those of us holding space for her, this is when we get goose bumps and can feel the creational, universal forces present in the room. There is a power, a strength, a primal, wild energy that is breath-taking.

Transformation is intense because:

- The duration of the surge is longer – 90 seconds.

- The surges are closer together, coming every 2–3 minutes.

- You are in the sensation for longer, with less time to recover in between.

There is now only a thin rim of cervix left holding the baby's head back, so the pressure is intense. This is a good thing, because it means it won't take long for that last little bit of cervix to melt away over the baby's head.

Other possible signs of transformation include shivering and sweating. You don't like it anymore: you want to go home, or go somewhere else if you are home. You want to come back and finish off another day, but you don't want to do anymore today. Your pain guides begin to shout, "What the heck is going on? Why is this happening?" You question how long you will be doing this labor thing. You might ask for pain medication, or vomit, or cry. You may feel more vulnerable and visible than you ever have before.

You have come to a bridge that only you can cross: one that is getting you from one mountain peak to the next, into another realm, an entirely new dimension. All your support people can cheer you on and encourage you, but it is you who has to put one foot in front of the other, one surge at a time, on that damn bridge that is shaking and so high in the air you're sure you'll die, and there is no turning back. What if you don't like the other dimension? What if motherhood is too much? The fear guides are now also shouting; our old friends "unworthy" and "incapable" will probably turn up. This is the blood and sweat and tears of transformation; this is the bridge, and only you can cross it.

Then, just like that, you are on the other side. Now, dear sister, your baby is just around another bend.

> "I think in every birth, despite all the very many ways that they unfold, there comes a singularly fragile moment of lucidity for the laboring mother. That moment is often met with an emotional deluge of vulnerability and fear; it explains why that moment can be so easily lost. To recognize that moment, that clear, calm and peaceful moment in a birthing mother is a call to those around her to respond to it in an equally clear, calm and peaceful way. My lucid moment came right at the end when all I could see in front of me was an episiotomy and ventouse. I got up, braced myself against my husband and despite all the odds and an unyielding 'strawberry', birthed my third son after 26 hours on the bedroom floor. Lucky for me, my midwife was there to catch him."
> Germaine, third baby, UK/Singapore

Good things to do in transformation include:

- Sound breathing – keep the sound *loooowwwww.*

- Movement – swaying, humming

- Try getting onto your hands and knees

- See if pressure or heat on your back/sacrum helps

- Let water calm you: get in the tub or shower

- Relax your jaw

- Think of a one-word mantra, like "open"

- Take sips of water from a straw

- Find a way to say yes instead of no

- Relax between the surges, letting your body be as limp and relaxed as possible

- Let the sensation be big, and find a way to flow with it

Note to birth companions: this is when your calm, reassuring presence is needed most. She probably won't let you out of her sight. You probably will be supporting her a lot with pressure on her sacrum or back, joining her in sound breathing so she can stay in touch with her breath, and encouraging her that she is nearly there: "You are so strong, and baby is almost here."

Labor and sexual trauma

Labor may trigger unwanted memories for a woman who has experienced any kind of sexual violence. It will be particularly important for her to feel safe, supported, and not forced in any way.

In these circumstances, I would recommend the following special measures:

- Choose a midwife as a PCP if possible.

- Share your previous trauma with your PCP during pregnancy – this is important because you want to ensure they take the time to gain your permission before doing any vaginal examinations or touching your body in any way, specifically with any force. They will also need to be more aware of their language, to avoid saying things like "Just relax and don't fight it, and you'll be fine."

- Ask yourself honestly if there is anything further you need to explore in your healing journey and consider finding qualified counsellors or hypnotherapists in your area.

- Elizabeth Davis is a midwife with a passion in the area of survivors and birth and you can find her online at www.elizabethdavis.com

Do

- Begin taking notice of your breath throughout the day, and breathing into your belly, your ribs, your diaphragm. Note when your breath becomes shallow and when you hold it. Breathing is your best friend in labor.

- Practice active relaxation and body scanning at night before sleeping: you are learning and practicing skills for lifelong health and stress management, not only birth.

- Build your support team to help you stay home for the early parts of labor.

- Join an empowering birth preparation class taught by an independent educator. If you don't have any in your area you can find good classes online, including the Love Based Birth class.

CHAPTER 16

Pain And The Tools To Cope

*"If you have access to create your own experience
would you create misery or pleasure?"*
Sadhguru, Indian mystic

One of the most common fears women have about birth is their ability and capacity to cope with the pain involved. This is not surprising, considering how many scary, horror-filled drama stories we hear from our sisters, neighbors, friends, and the way the media loves to portray birth as something to be feared. Let's explore all we can to get into a better position (pun intended) to understand, manage and use our labor pain as a guide helping us create a love-filled birth.

Firstly, fear of pain is normal, and pain – or at least 'strong sensations' (not every woman describes them as pain) – is an important part of the process. I warn couples who come to my class that if they are looking for the class that teaches them how to have a pain-free birth, they are in the wrong room. We all laugh.

The good news is that pain, just like fear, is also a productive and useful guide. We want to start shifting our mindset to see it as a force that makes us proactive: enroll in a gentle birth preparation class, join prenatal yoga, and practice ways to relax.

Every other experience of pain in the body happens when something is not right. Maybe you broke your leg, your appendix burst, you ate something that gave you terrible gas pain, recovered from surgery, got a tattoo…The pain always has purpose; it is there to guide us to do something about it, to find help. It fires up our fight-or-flight response, and the nervous system screams "Get help!" At the same time, adrenaline and other stress hormones move blood to the periphery of our bodies (we want that extra oxygen in our arms and legs to run and fight), shorten our breath, and increase our heart rate.

When that happens in labor, you will need to reassure your pain guide: "Thanks for the warning, but we are not going anywhere. Everything is OK. I was expecting this; we are having a baby." In labor, the purpose of the pain guide is to prompt you to get out of your bed, move, sway, breathe, moan, lean against a warm body like your partner, reach out to hold a loving hand, or get under the shower. Those movements and activities have two purposes:

1. They help you to relax and cope, to reduce the intensity of the sensation.

2. They help your baby to find its way through the birth maze.

In my prenatal yoga class, my teacher Morgan loves to guide us to notice the difference between being stationary like a statue and using movement to cope with the intensity of doing one-minute wide-legged goddess squats on repeat. We hold this position for a minute without movement, and then we pause and stretch and then hold for another minute, softening, swaying and finding movement, breathing and flowing to be with the intensity. The difference is incredible, try it.

If you don't have access to an awesome prenatal yoga teacher like Morgan, there are some videos available on LoveBasedBirth.com you can use for your own practice.

There are two factors that will affect the degree to which you experience a labor surge:

1. your internal environment and

2. your external environment.

Your internal environment

The idea here is simple; the more tension you hold in your muscles, the more pain you will experience. Remember the fear, tension, pain syndrome from chapter 7?

Imagine someone who doesn't like the dentist – who carries dental trauma from a previous experience. When they walk into the surgery, smell that smell of lidocaine and toothpaste, sit down in that chair and get reclined, their nervous system is in full fight-or-flight mode: "How do I get out of here?" Their adrenaline and other stress hormones are shooting through the roof, their jaw is clenched and their pupils dilated – and nothing has even happened yet!

How do you think that cleaning or filling will go?

Now instead, imagine someone who doesn't mind the dentist, who has always had good experiences, who likes a chance to sit in the waiting room cruising the magazines and is happy to be lowered in the chair, knowing that it will give them a chance to do some mental planning for their upcoming holiday.

How will they experience that cleaning or filling?

All our previous experiences and exposures create our reality. That is why it's so important to make a priority of discovering the hidden influences on you and your beliefs around birth long before you are in the thick of it.

Shifting the mindset

How can we embrace the idea of pain, not as enemy, but as guide? Your birth guide wants to be your friend, someone you can rely on to get you to where you want to go. I urge you to learn how to work with this powerful force and understand how your thoughts can influence your body's response to pain, by considering pain as the following:

P – Purposeful: bringing your baby into your arms

A – Anticipated: you have time to plan for it; you are expecting to meet it

I – Intermittent: not constant, but coming and going as required

N – Normal: your body is in a state of health; you are having a baby!

Note: The fact that surges are 'intermittent' is a big deal. Milli Hill, author of *The Positive Birth Book* did the maths for us and discovered in an average 8-hour labor, a woman can expect to be 'in pain' for only around 23% of the time. The other 77% is 'pain free' because she will be between surges.

All the tools described in Section 1 are powerful ways to increase your coping abilities and work with your pain guides including:

- Addressing fears
- Breath
- Visualizations
- Affirmations
- Guided meditation
- Understanding the mind/body connection
- Sound breathing
- Water
- Upright positions or hands and knees
- Safe environments
- Loving support

Can we find joy in running a marathon or climbing a mountain? We can when we decide to meet the challenges along the way with a joyful acceptance.

"I was surprised my birth was neither painful or tiring."
Nicole, third baby, Singapore

The external environment

The birthing environment is so crucial, because even mild anxiety caused by the external environment (remember, oxytocin doesn't love strangers, lights or commotion, but adrenaline and stress hormones do) can spark the body into a state of fight or flight and stress. The mind doesn't know the difference between real and imagined, and will just create the hormones needed to match whatever it 'thinks' is going on.

The baby's position

Another environmental factor that can affect the level of pain experienced in birth is baby's position. While there are many factors that affect the baby's position, the best position is considered to be with

- head downwards.
- baby's back on the left side, looking towards Mum's opposite hip
- chin tucked onto chest;
- hands out of the way – hands on heart

This is a good image to work with, which we touched on in Chapter 7.

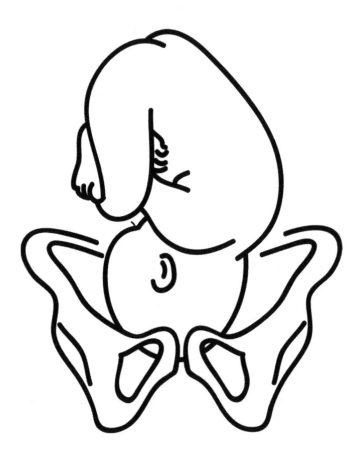

Starting from 30–32 weeks of your pregnancy, make it your priority to know what position your little one is in; have your PCP show you how to feel your belly and identify the position. You can find more information of how to palpate your own belly on the Love Based Birth website.

·······
Do
·······

- Take time prenatally and as early as possible to start learning more about your own relationship with pain, and then collect and practice tools that will help you surrender to your body's sensations.

- Get friendly with your pain guides.

- Explore these questions: what are the other times in your life you have felt pain in your body? What were the circumstances around that? How did you cope?

- Find out where and how your baby is positioned and keep track of it for yourself.

CHAPTER 17

....

Everything Water

*"People never sing...except in the bathroom. Birthing women also
make their natural sounds next to running bath water.
There is something about the power of water.
People are drawn to water, spas, and sacred streams.
Women in labor are drawn to water, too."*
Michel Odent MD, obstetrician, author

Water is an element that promotes relaxation, and relaxation is just what we need during labor.

When I was having panic attacks, I discovered that one of the best ways to ride them out was to get in the shower, specifically, in the shower with my head directly under the shower head. The noise would drown out the screaming in my head, the water would beautifully blend with the waterfalls coming from my eyes and nose, and the sensation of the falling water would give other sensations for my mind/body to notice. Eventually the hyperventilation would slow, and I would find and calm my breath, and it would take me the rest of the way back to shore.

Water is therapeutic

Water is nutrition during pregnancy, so take weekly (at least) Epsom salt baths, stay hydrated, and swim as much as you can. If you live somewhere where water is scarce, get creative with your bath water. When you use Epsom salts, you don't need any soaps or shampoos, so the water can be used for multiple family members. You can also use it to water your plants for that week (Epsom salt is a natural plant fertilizer), wash your floors, or wash your car!

> "I swam so much during my pregnancy as part of my exercise regime and physical preparation – it felt appropriate to be in the water, breathe below and above it, and birth my baby from one water medium into another."
> Anonymous, first baby, Singapore

Here are three ways you can use water in labor:

1. In early labor, run yourself an Epsom salt bath, turn out all the lights and tune into your body, breath and bath. The Epsom salts will help you to relax and soothe your muscles.

2. A warm water bottle on your belly or lower back can be used during all stages of labor.

3. A warm shower: sit on a stool or an exercise ball and let the water flow down your back. If you have a handheld showerhead, ask your birth partner or birth supporter to direct it onto your lower back. A warm shower is appropriate during all stages of labor, and best during rock and roll and transformation.

> "During labor, it was so relaxing to just sit in the shower on my hands and knees and let the water hit my lower back."
> Kyra, first baby, America/Singapore

4. Birth pool or bathtub: let the water take weight off your ligaments and joints. You can used them early labor, or hold off until rock and roll and transformation, so that you have something to look forward to when things get more intense.

5. Drink it! Hydration is key to helping your uterine muscles work in harmony. Coconut water is a perfect electrolyte drink for labor; it will refuel your muscles and keep leg cramps away.

Birth in water

In my home birth practice, about 80% of the births I attend are in water. In the several hundred water births I have attended, there have been only two women that I can remember who got in, couldn't get comfortable, and got out, deciding water wasn't their thing. The more common reaction is a sigh of relief as their bodies become buoyant. I usually get a nasty look when I suggest it might be time to get out to pee. I can't tell you how many women get out to pee and then nearly run back from the toilet to the bath.

> "During my surges at the beginning, the hot water from the shower helped the pain. In the end, when we were in the birthing tub at the hospital, it helped the pain and helped so that I didn't tear, and also I think it helped my son come out much easier."
> Jasmine, first baby, UK/Singapore

The idea of using water, besides the relaxation element, is that it is a gentle start for the baby. Because they have been in water, in the amniotic sac, for nine months, coming from the mother's body to land in another water world can be less stressful.

What are the benefits of water birth?

Benefits for mother

- Water is soothing, comforting, and relaxing.
- Buoyancy: your body becomes lighter and feels freer in movement.

"I remember the moment that (my midwife) looked at me and said I was ready to get in the birthing pool. There was this elated feeling that I must be getting close to meeting my baby! Those next few hours were timeless. The warm water embraced me gently, giving buoyancy to my body and easing the intensity of the surges. I loved the feeling of my legs slightly floating and being able to keep my hands centimeters from my belly, energetically feeling Baby through the water. And in its own way, the birthing pool made me feel that I had gone back to my mother's womb in order to access my own. As I started to birth my baby, it was incredible to me that she waited patiently between surges with her head under water, eyes closed, until the next surge brought her shoulders and body out of my opened vagina and straight into my own hands. She had gone from water to water, and the transition was so smooth that she could wait for more than a minute for her shoulders and body to follow. What a beautiful entry into this world."

Amber first baby, USA/Singapore

- Relaxation: because you are more relaxed, your surges will be more effective, the muscle better oxygenated, and you will also be able to breathe more deeply, providing better oxygenation for the baby.

- Resting more deeply between surges helps to conserve energy.

- Water gives you a space all to yourself, like a protective bubble. It is much harder for your PCP to *do* things to you like put their fingers inside your vagina while you are breathing baby down, cut an episiotomy, or make any other of the mostly unnecessary interventions.

- Water's privacy bubble also supports the release of oxytocin.

- Physical relaxation supports mental relaxation; when the mind isn't as busy, it is easier for you to "get in the zone" and surrender your birthing body to the process.

- Water can lower raised blood pressure caused by stress or anxiety.

- Lowering stress and anxiety by finding more relaxation and ease increases your body's ability to release more endorphins – the pain relief hormones.

- Water provides natural lubrication, and as you will generally be more relaxed and so will your perineum, so the chances of tearing are reduced.

> "I had a very rapid birth with my daughter and only managed to get into the tub for about five minutes before she was born. Those five minutes were bliss; they coincided with me being fully dilated and about to bring her down. I felt that the water slowed things down enough so that I could breathe and rest, even though it was for a short time. Then birthing her into the water was wonderful, as it was warm and comforting, and I think acted as a very good pain reliever for her crowning and birth.
> Miranda, second baby, New Zealand/Singapore

Benefits for baby

- Water makes for an easy transition: from water into water. Water babies are noted to be more relaxed at birth, often still curled up and almost asleep.

- Water reduces the opportunity for the PCP to manipulate the baby for the birth of the shoulders, and increases the chance of a "hands off" birth.

Disadvantages of water

We are learning more about the microbiome and the importance of baby picking up these good bacteria on the way out of the vagina. It is natural to wonder what effect, if any, the water has on the microbiome. To date, there haven't been any studies that I am aware of on this topic.

Not all PCPs are comfortable with water, and some want to get mums out immediately after the birth. This disrupts those first minutes after birth when mother and baby are meeting for the first time. Often PCPs insist the cord is cut first, depriving the baby of its blood. Be sure to discuss with your PCP what their policy is.

> "I liked it a lot. I would have loved to give birth in water but due to a previous C-section, my PCP did not allow it."
> Anonymous, second baby, France/Singapore(VBAC)

Note: Water temperature is important. If you are soaking in a tub, it should be at around body temperature: 35–36 degrees. You don't want it too hot in early labor/labor, or you will sweat too much and become dehydrated, or raise your own body temperature. And for birth, you don't want it to be too hot for the baby. It should be slightly cooler than the amniotic fluid was (your body temperature, 37 degrees).

Waters opening

"My waters broke" or "my water ruptured": both statements sound so violent. Who wants to feel like something is breaking or rupturing inside their body? Not me! Much of the language around birth can be softened and made more positive. I prefer the term 'waters opening' or 'releasing', and I encourage you to make this vocabulary shift.

A dad recently came up to me after our class about labor, very excited to tell me, "Red, you busted open a myth I have always had until today. I thought waters always opened first. That is what happens in all of the Bollywood movies!"

Statistically speaking, waters open as a first sign of labor only in about 20% of pregnancies. The most common time for them to open is during transformation or breathing the baby down, because the internal pressure is highest at this point. Environment and nutrition can affect the integrity of the water bag, increasing your chances of it opening early if you live in a very polluted city or have a diet lacking whole foods, vegetables and fruits. If that is the case, consider taking 500 mg of a good vitamin C supplement daily.

Once your water opens, you are on a time clock, because there is no longer a sterile field protecting baby, so bacteria can climb upwards, causing infection in the uterus. There is a vast range of protocols PCPs use, from immediate induction to waiting for several days.

Be well informed to make decisions and have a dialogue with your PCP –This is what you need to be aware of when your waters open:

- Check to see the color when they open – they should be clear. Green or brown waters are a reason to check in with your PCP right away (see below).

- Check in with your baby right away when your waters release. It will be a change of pressure for them, so they might be surprised. Ask how they are doing and reassure them that it means they are on the way, and you are ready.

- You should be in the environment where you are most relaxed and likely to go into labor on your own. Don't allow any vaginal examinations if your waters have opened and you are not in labor! –Nothing much will be discovered and it increases your risk of infection.

- Antibiotics are often recommended after 24 hours.

- Waters opening as a first sign of labor is not reason on its own for healthy babies to be separated from their mothers or be taken to the NICU routinely after birth

Opening the water bag manually

Opening the water bag manually is a very common intervention. PCPs like to do it for two main reasons: to speed up labor, and to see if there is meconium (baby's poo) in the water.

Opening the water bag can make labor go quicker because rather than the cushion of the water bag dilating the cervix, the harder baby's head will be doing a better job. Likewise, if the waters haven't yet opened, it is impossible to know if they are clear or have meconium in them.

However, it is important to keep in mind, that every action has a reaction, and your baby is not a silent passenger. He is in there, moving and shifting and solving a huge problem – how do I get out of this tight, squeezing place?

The possible negative outcomes of opening the water bag are:

- The baby gets his head stuck in an unfavorable position. When the waters were poked open, he might have been turning his head to one side, maybe by only a couple of degrees, trying another angle to come down at. If the water cushion, which made it easier to rotate his head, rushes out at that moment, he could settle incorrectly, causing labor to go on even longer and possibly not end with a vaginal exit.

- It sets the clock ticking – especially if it's done in the early part of labor. Opening the water bag is one of the interventions that there is no returning from, because we can't take it back or turn it off.

Except in rare circumstances, this intervention is not needed. Babies know when it is a good time for them to open their own bags.

Meconium

Meconium is your baby's first poo. It is black and sticky and like tar. Interestingly, it is thick and sticky for a good reason: it helps to keep the intestines open so the walls don't grow together during gestation.

Your baby usually has a clenched bottom to keep the meconium in. Unclenching and letting out the meconium can happen for two different reasons:

1. A sudden startle or stress causes them to relax their anal sphincters.

2. Maturity –beyond 40 weeks' gestation their little bottom sphincters naturally relax; they just become tired of holding.

How meconium-stained fluid is managed varies vastly from PCP to PCP. However, meconium on its own, without other signs of fetal distress, is not an indication for a Caesarean.

Couples often ask me, "If the evidence for best practice is so well documented, why doesn't every practitioner follow the same practice? It makes no sense." True, but it is complicated, especially because the protocols are often not even set by medical research or senior hospital staff, but by the hospital's insurance company – think malpractice insurance.

CASE STUDY

I recently worked with a woman who had put a lot of effort into preparing for a gentle birth. She hired a doula and found a PCP whose philosophy matched her own. She arrived at the hospital fully dilated to discover her chosen PCP was out of town; there was a junior filling in. She was breathing her baby down beautifully; the baby was nice and relaxed on the heart rate monitor, but when her waters opened and the junior saw the meconium staining, he insisted on an emergency Caesarean. He silenced her protests with, "Do you want your baby to die?" And off she went for a, probably unnecessary, Caesarean with the baby's head already visible. The baby cried immediately, was strong and healthy and did not show any signs of fetal distress or respiratory issues.

Babies born in their water bags

Sometimes the waters do not open at all during labor or birth. Some babies are born still inside their bags; it is called 'in the caul'. Our ancestors considered being born in the caul as auspicious: a sign that a great leader was coming into the community. It is something very magical to see; there are many photos and videos you can see on the internet if you type "birth in caul" (again, be careful with your internet cruising). There are also photos and videos on the Love Based Birth website if you search "birth in the caul".

CASE STUDY
I had a magical birth recently with a third-time mum. She labored quietly in the early morning hours in the birth pool with her husband gently encouraging her, and the kids sleeping in the next room. When her baby emerged, we were surprised to see it facing up to us (posterior) – he had been anterior for the last weeks leading up to birth. The baby was still in the amniotic sac. What an incredible sight! As he paused there looking up at us, through the bag and through the water, waiting for the next surge to birth the rest of his body, time stood still. It was as if another dimension had opened, and we could see for just a moment how thin is the curtain separating worlds and realities.

Do

- Consider how you will use water during labor and birth.

- If your PCP offers a water birthing service, ask specific questions about their protocols.

- Visualize those crystal-clear waters surrounding your baby.

....

CHAPTER 18

Birth Partners

"When you love someone, the best thing you can offer is your presence. How can you love if you are not there?"
Thich Nhat Hanh Zen Master, author, peace activist

Having a loving presence at the birth is an essential ingredient for a laboring woman – a loving presence that allows her to be who she needs to be and do what she needs to; one that does not try to control her or have any agenda other than a willingness to be her witness. As her lover, *you* are the best person to support her during this time of transformation. Your role is key. In this chapter, I have given some general guidelines that will help you understand the basic needs of a laboring woman.

You are also going to have a powerful experience yourself: you will be right there, a crucial part of something incredibly big and powerful. You will feel helpless or powerless at times, completely euphoric and ecstatic at others. After the birth, you might feel like you failed her somehow; you might have layers of guilt or grief at not having been able to stop something from happening, or from witnessing something difficult. You might feel completely overwhelmed by the experience of becoming a parent. This is all normal.

So it's also important to have your own support structure, to be able to share your experience of how it was for *you*. If you are with an independent midwife, she will likely ask you at one of the postnatal visits if there is anything about the birth that you want to share or talk about. I'd invite you to go for it: if there is anything you are unsure about, concerned about, didn't understand, or want to say, take advantage of the opportunity. You might find your feeling about, or experience of, the birth is very different from that of your partner – this would be completely normal too.

If you are preparing for your second or third baby, I highly recommend taking the opportunity to explore the previous experiences and the possible fears or doubts that you are carrying from them, and clearing out all those cobwebs so they don't come into this next birth with you.

Partner experiences

One of my favorite aspects of what I do is 'debriefing' birth with couples. Often it happens years after the birth, when they are preparing for the next baby. It doesn't matter how much time has passed, I find both sides have lingering feelings to explore. Sometimes they are strong and on the surface, or they may be stuck and take some digging to find.

CASE STUDIES

Recently, in a birth preparation session, a couple talked about their 'express train' birth the first time around – an unplanned home birth. The last part of the labor was so fast that the baby came out onto the bathroom floor, with no one in attendance but the dad. When the mum described the experience, she was glowing. She was so proud of how calm and relaxed she remained through the labor, how she managed to do it completely on her own without external intervention or assistance. She wanted another home birth, this time a planned one.

Dad was traumatized by the experience, though. The prospect of another, home birth – even a planned one – was overwhelming for him, and he was pushing for a hospital birth instead. He said he didn't want to risk being in that position of total responsibility again.

Having the ability to discuss their feelings while someone witnessed them and reflected back helped them to remove the layers of separation they had so they could come to a decision about the place of birth that felt good for both of them.

Another couple, preparing for their second baby, shared their story. During the first birth, Mum was doing fabulously with her labor; she was a 'cat in the closet' kind of laborer – liked everything quiet, didn't want to be touched and was very sensitive to noise. (This is quite common, especially for women who are not in fear but in their own flow.) This dad wanted to help, and he thought he was helping by talking to her, encouraging her, massaging her shoulders, asking her questions like whether she was OK and whether she wanted to go to the hospital yet. However, that was annoying to her, she kept shushing him and eventually waved him out of the room. He felt rejected and thought he wasn't needed, so he went and lay on the couch and took a nap. How did Mum feel? Abandoned.

They were both carrying those feelings – rejection, confusion, abandonment, anger – around two years later, when preparing for the next baby.

In our session, she had the opportunity to explain to him how important it was to her that he was there with her, that he didn't leave her alone. She wanted him to be near and available, she just didn't want him to talk or fidget or try to fix anything. She didn't want him 'in the container' with her, distracting her focus; instead she wanted him just outside it, ensuring that the container was safe and free from distractions. Once they heard each other, they both felt relieved and ready to look forward to the next birth. Dad knew he was needed and had a better idea of what to do for her; and Mum was happy that he did want to play that role.

Communication

When planning your baby's birth together, get clear about roles and expectations. To be frank, most women want their lovers to be their 'knights in shining armor' during birth, but that rarely happens unless everyone is well prepared and roles have been established.

The way to do this is for the birthing woman to communicate clearly what she anticipates wanting from her partner; her partner – you – need to hear what her expectation is and let her know if that is something you are keen to, or able to fulfill.

> "I feel as though my husband's presence was vital to my birth. In that moment, I needed him. I just needed his attention and presence. His hands on my body was what comforted me the most. I wouldn't let him leave my side."
> Amanda, first baby, USA/Singapore

And be prepared for it to change. The women who think they will want tons of touch in labor end up not wanting it, and vice versa. As birth support people, we have to be willing to go with whatever turns up, and be flexible in the moment. Like everything in life, the clearer the communication, the better. And we will never get it exactly right, and that is ok, too.

> "He was fully supportive and adoring of my birth plan. But beyond that, he had minimal involvement, which in my mind now, is how it should be. It's a deeply feminine experience. He was there as a deeply masculine energy – he was quiet, watchful, protective but he stayed out of it. That was exactly what he needed to do, and what I needed him to do. I wanted to birth alone, be with my power, but his total commitment to my vision and support on the side lines (and willingness to jump in if I called for him) was right for us."
> Caroline, second baby UK/Singapore

I attended a birth recently, where Mum was in rock and roll labor and Dad was sitting on the floor nearby, quietly supporting and eating a bag of chips.

There was the rustling bag, crunching, more bag-rustling and then suddenly, "Get out of here with that!" So off he went and barely came back. From my many conversations with her, I knew how much she wanted her man to be there and to be present with her. She wanted it more than anything. However, the concentration she required in those moments, to work with her body's power, didn't allow space for an unconsciously produced distraction.

A crash course on presence

1. Find a good combination of being fully available and fully invisible.

   Many midwives knit during labor; it is quiet, keeps them occupied, but less occupied than reading a book. It gives a message something like, "I am here if you need anything; I am fully in this with you, but you can take your time. I'm fine and have nowhere else to be." Depending on the woman, sitting and staring at her can make her feel she needs to perform, or hurry.

   You don't have to take up knitting, but try to practice how to sit back and simply 'be available'. It's a bit of an art!

2. Turn your phone off.

   In our busy, connected world, I hear frequently from frustrated mums who felt angry because their partner was on the phone while they labored. This gave them the impression that checking emails, cruising Facebook, or playing games was more important than being involved in what was happening.

   Treat this like the most important business meeting you have ever been in, with two owners discussing a merger. You are only required to be present to witness all that's going on, and to contribute verbally or physically as requested, depending on how the meeting unfolds. Using a phone in such a situation would be considered impolite, unless there was an emergency or during an agreed break. It's about respect.

3. Don't talk during surges (I'm generalizing).

   She needs her full focus to stay with the sensation she is experiencing. She is concentrating on her breath and going on a deep exploration of herself. When we talk, we take her out of her zone. There is an exception during the transformation stage, when verbal encouragement will likely be required with every surge if she is finding it hard to cope. "You are almost there. You are doing great. One surge at a time."

4. Offer, don't ask.

   When we ask a question, we stimulate the neocortex, that front part of the brain that has nothing to do with birth. As labor advances, women move further and further into their instinctive brain, which is where we want them to be, so we try not to distract that. Seeing her in that instinctual, primal place might make you find her incredibly attractive during labor.

   An example of offer rather then ask is rather than asking, "Are you thirsty?" or "Would you like some water?", try, after every couple of surges, put the glass with a straw in her range and say, "Take a sip."

What to do when

In early labor your job is to provide reassurance and distraction, ensure she stays hydrated – and time the surges.

You don't need to time every surge! It is not possible to be present if you are timing and writing down every single surge for hours. . Just check what the surges are doing when something changes – when you start to notice that they are more intense or closer together.

Otherwise, forget about the time, put away the contraction timing app, or your watch, and stay present.

The only reason you care about what the surges are doing is if you need to report to your midwife who is not there yet, or if you are wondering if it is time to go to your birth place. If your midwife is there or you're already at your birth place, forget all about timing surges timing; others have that covered for you.

Arriving at the hospital

If you are planning birth at a hospital, remember, you want to get there to have your baby, not hang around for hours or days. Ideally, you are getting there in rock and roll labor.

This means mum will be moving slowly, stopping each time she has a surge to breathe and lean up against something, perhaps you. Walk slowly and breathe yourself. Don't try to rush her anywhere. Refuse the wheelchair the hospital security might offer. The walk to the labor suite will do her good, and the wheelchair has an energy that is very different from hers, as a strong, a powerful laboring woman.

The logistics will differ depending on what country you are in. Ideally, you have pre-registered and/or can go straight up to delivery suite and register after the baby is born.

Settling into your room

Once in the labor suite, stay with her while they do all the initial checks – blood pressure, temperature, baby's heart, probably a vaginal examination to check how far dilated she is. (Generally, if she is under 3cm dilated, it is a good idea to go back home. Getting up to 5 cm can take time when it is not an 'express train' birth.)

It is very valuable if you answer all the questions for her so she can just stay focused and in "the zone". Remember, her job is to work with her body, and your job is to maintain a safe undisturbed space. You do all the interactions with the hospital staff and look after all the details. She breathes and moves.

The kind of questions you'll be asked when you check in include:

- What time did her contractions start?
- Are her waters opened?
- What was the last thing she ate?
- Is she allergic to any medications, foods or anything else?
- How many weeks is she/what is her estimated due date?
- Who is your doctor/midwife/care provider?

Find out all those things beforehand, so you don't have to say, "Sorry babe, but do you have any drug allergies?" in the middle of a surge.

At this point, ask who the head nurse in charge of your room is and give her your birth plan (the one signed by your doctor).

Once all the initial checks are done, go up to the nurses' station and thank them for their wonderful help, tell them how excited you are, and what type of support you are looking for. For example, if you live in a country where they love to ask the 'pain score', please tell them that won't be necessary in your room. (The pain scale runs from 0 to 10. Asking a laboring woman to focus on the pain and give it a number is completely inappropriate. The next question is probably "Are you ready for your epidural now?") Say, "You can ask my partner how you can help make her more comfortable, but please don't ask how much pain she is in." You might also want to add that you have been practicing gentle birthing, relaxation techniques, and that you would like to keep things dim and quiet, and avoid all unnecessary distractions.

Do your best to find a balance somewhere between kind and assertive; being rude or demanding will get you no-where. If you have done your homework, it should be easier, because you will have picked a doctor and hospital that are in favor of natural birth and used to all these requests.

Roles

In a hospital setting, these are some of the roles the birth companion will fill:

Gatekeeper

In the gatekeeper role you must stay by her side so she can feel you safe guarding her birth space; talk with nurses and handle visitors. You are the buffer between the medical staff and the laboring woman. Ideally, and unless there are special circumstances, get the nurses to come to you first before they disturb labor, when they want to take blood pressure, listen to baby, and so on.

> "He took care of everything and I could fully focus on delivering: he decorated the room, he was point of contact with the nurses, he gave me drinks and food, he massaged, gave me warming pillow, motivated me."
> Anonymous, VBAC, Singapore

Interior decorator

You need to take care of all the details, so the only thing mum has to do is work with her laboring body.

Take the initiative long before labor to check out the birth bag and know where everything is. (She might want you to get in the shower with her, so pack some shorts for yourself if you'll be in a hospital or birth center.) She shouldn't have to direct you around the birth bag at the same time as laboring. You need to set up the music, keep the lights dim, hang a sign on the door.

Offer all three levels of support: emotional, mental and physical.

- Physical: offer her water and remind her to use the toilet, use warm packs, touch her gently, do light touch massage if she likes it or sacral pressure, breathe with her, smooth her forehead with a washcloth, bring her what she needs. Remember to offer rather than ask. Be present.

> "He helped me to the bathroom and held me when I needed to walk back and forth. He wasn't intrusive, [he] let me ask him for help."
> Kelly, 1st baby, America

- Emotional: as labor progresses, tell her you love her, remind her she is another step closer to having your beloved baby in her arms, say things like: "you're doing beautifully", continue to look for ways to comfort her. Be present. Put your phone away.

> "There wasn't one thing. His presence was so huge for me, though. I would just look at him and see how much he loved me in his eyes, and how much he wanted to help. He was my greatest support and our birth is one of our favourite memories."
> Kyra, first baby, America/Singapore

- Mental: gently remind her of the visualizations you know she has been practicing, remind her of her strength and power, and the other things she has done in the past, do sound breathing with her. Be present; but be ready to be completely quiet and give her space, as well. That might be what works best for her. Remember she might want to birth like a 'cat in a closet'.

You might want to write yourself a reminder card with something along the lines of:

I will remind myself to

- offer her water/coconut water between surges;

- be ready to give whatever physical support she needs: sacral pressure, hip squeeze, light touch and more;

- be OK with silence and not being physically needed;

- give her space to do it her way;

- take care of all the details for her;

- encourage her to empty her bladder (hourly) and spend some surges on the toilet;

- suggest using water: a warm shower (put the exercise ball or stool in the shower for her) or bath, or a hot water bottle.

- breathe with her – you know what specific practices work best for her; generally this is belly breathing, slow and deep

- join in sound breathing (deep and low) during rock and roll and transformation stages, if it feels like it helps and she needs companionship/focus ; and

- walk with her, sing with her, dance with her.

Don't forget to hydrate and eat yourself, so you keep your stamina up as well!

Partner affirmations for birth

Affirmations are useful for you too. I encourage you to play with something like the list below. Find three or four that make sense to you and write them out or put them in your phone so you can refer to them daily/weekly.

You can add her name or the baby's name to each of them, to make them more concrete and personal, or just say, my partner/my wife/my love", whatever feels most comfortable.

- I desire joy to be a continuous feeling, (my partner's name) and I experience during pregnancy, birth and post birth.
- I desire that our baby (baby name) feels and connects with us in a way that makes him/her feel loved and safe.
- I love the way (my partner's name) body is growing; she is radiant.
- I love and support my partner on this incredible journey.
- I am a compassionate, loving, caring and adoring father and partner.
- I am patient with my partner.
- I will always be there for my partner and our baby/(baby name).
- I will listen to my partner and be attentive to her needs.
- Our baby/(name) is growing and developing just as it should.
- Our baby hears my spoken or silent voice, and is already connected to me.
- I am ready, receptive and extremely grateful to become a father.
- I understand that our baby is a separate individual, and I give him/her enough space for his/her individuality.
- I see the world through the eyes of our baby and participate in his/her sense of wonder and joy.
- Our baby feels my love.
- Our life is in perfect balance.
- I welcome our baby with joy and love and an open heart.
- I have love for all my children.

- I love our baby, and our baby loves me.

- I love my partner, and my partner loves our baby and me.

- I make decisions for my baby that are for the greatest good for them and everyone involved.

- Our baby feels my calm and relaxed presence.

- Our baby is safe and secure at all times.

- Our baby is healthy.

- I am experiencing great love.

> "He talked me out of my misery with a relaxation exercise. I was saying that I wanted a C-section, that this was too much pain because I still wasn't getting closer to 3-minute contractions (more like 6-minute contractions) and I thought I had so much more to go. I thought that I was still in early labor, whereas my husband said I was going into transition. He reminded me I wanted a natural birth and distracted me from the intense pain with a creative relaxation visualization that helped to calm me down a lot."
> Catherine, first baby, Singapore

Choose from this list to start your affirmation:

I acknowledge	I desire	I trust
I affirm	I enjoy	I will
I allow	I follow	In every-way
I am	I fully accept	In this moment
I choose	I make	Right now I
I connect	I own	Today I
I create	I realise	Yes, I

- Follow it up with what you want to express.

- Then add this insurance statement to the end of your affirmation:

  - I experience this or something better.

  - Please make this for the highest good for me, [partner name] and our baby and for everyone involved.

....
Do
....

- Put in the effort to learn how best to support the labor process.

- Understand that you don't need to take the pain or intensity away, or make something better, you just need to be present and available.

- Anticipate her needs.

- Be patient with yourself.

- Recognize the importance of your role.

- Write and use your own affirmations.

CHAPTER 19

Birth

"Experience of the phenomenal capacity of our birthing body can give us an enduring sense of our own power as women. Birth is the beginning of life, the beginning of mothering, and of fathering. We all deserve a good beginning."

Sarah J. Buckley MD, author

It is common to feel a great sense of relief once your body is fully dilated, maybe because the sensations change, and the surges return to the pre-transformation pattern, or maybe because you know you are almost finished.

As an observer of birth, I see that the opening phase is all about being passive, finding ways to relax into what is happening. Once baby starts moving down, however, there is an energy shift. Women get more present in their surroundings; the actual birth part seems to require another type of connection.

When a woman in labor asks me, "How much longer, Red?" I often put it back to her saying, "I don't know. Can you feel your baby's head yet?" When there is no fear, when there is no shame, putting your fingers into your vagina to see if you can feel a head is normal and instinctual. It is also normal to have a feel when the baby is moving down to check on the process. Having this level of connection to what is happening gives a great sense of purpose and motivation, both very necessary when nearing any finish line. You become your own guide, with your breath and your internal process.

> "(I was surprised most by)how much I actually enjoyed the rawness of pushing and shouting. And how all the intense feelings just disappeared when I got the head of the baby out."
> Catherine, first baby, Singapore

Someone once told me (after we been through a birth together) that the only thing I could possibly do that was more intimate with a couple, besides being a home birth midwife, was sitting at the end of the bed while they made love. I agree! Birth is very intimate; it is sexual. It is same part of the body, the same hormones.

I showed a birth video today in my birth preparation class of an awesome birth I attended last year. The very well-prepared first-time mum felt her own baby's crown in the water, guided her out, caught her, and, brought her up out of the water to her chest. You don't see me at all because I was just outside of the camera frame, ready if she or the baby needed my help, just where I think PCPs belong most of the time.

After the video ended, one of the dads in the group asked in amazement, "She did that completely on her own. Is that common?" Yes, I stopped 'catching' babies some years back. I still do on the odd occasion of course, but most births I attend either the mum receives the baby or the dad/other parent does. What could be more special than your baby receiving her first touch from *your* loving hands?

> "Baby – The first thing I felt from my mum was being welcomed by her caressing my hair while I was still making my way out."
> Bea, third baby, Germany/Singapore

Connecting with the process of birth by physically feeling your body doing the work is especially helpful for survivors of sexual violence. It reminds us birth is not something that happens *to you*; it is something that *you do*.

Here are two myths that need dispelling:

1. Your PCP needs to 'deliver' your baby. Instinct governs nature, and your baby is no different. It knows how to birth itself. It is rare when anyone besides you needs to do much to receive the baby.

2. You need to push long and hard to get your baby out.

Your uterus will help you. It has a built-in ejection reflex that pushes baby down and out for you. While birthing a baby takes effort in an upright position, for a relaxed mum with a gentle care provider, it can feel more like an uncontrollable natural force of the body (think the last time you had diarrhea or vomiting) than something that you need to get into a mechanical rhythm with, like holding your breath while someone counts to 10 for you.

> "I was most surprised when my body started 'pushing' my baby out all on its own. My body completely took over and did what it needed to do."
>
> Amanda, first baby, America/Singapore (breech)

And here are two practices you should not have done to you unless it's a true emergency (someone's life is at risk):

1. Fundal pressure

    Fundal pressure is when someone pushes down on the top of your belly (uterus) to help eject the baby. It can cause the baby to become stressed as the pressure on the head intensifies, a higher chance of baby needing to be separated from you and spend time in intensive care after birth, postpartum hemorrhage because the uterus is in shock, uterine prolapse, bladder damage, perineal and pelvic floor damage, and it is especially dangerous for a VBAC birth as it increases the chance of uterine rupture.

2. Episiotomy

In an episiotomy scissors are used to cut the vaginal opening so there is more room for the baby to come out. It can cause more pain in recovery; long-term weakness in the pelvic floor, possibly leading to incontinence; prolapse (falling) of the bladder, uterus or bowel; and possible long-term pain during sexual penetration.

Note: There is a myth in Asia that Asian women are smaller "down there" so they need episiotomies at birth, a myth I have even read printed in hospital reading material here in Singapore. The reality is that Asian women also have smaller babies than western women, so if 'smaller' is true then it balances out. There are plenty of Asian women giving birth outside Asia without routine episiotomies. Don't let your PCP bully you with that statement. Find someone else to support you.

In 2012, a Cochrane Systematic Review collated the results of all the randomized controlled trials involving more than 5,000 women, and it showed significant benefits to restricting episiotomies. http://onlinelibrary.wiley.com/doi/10.1002/14651858.CD000081.pub2/abstract

These are both dangerous practices still done routinely by many PCPs. Like all interventions, they have a place and can be life-saving, without a doubt. But assuming women's bodies don't work and using them as routine is an insult.

After the baby is born

What does a holistic, immediate postpartum period (the first few hours after the birth) look like? "Motherbaby dyad" care, is the best and it simply means viewing the mother and baby as an inseparable unit and causing as little disturbance as possible to them, supporting the crucial time for bonding and attachment.

Most medical professionals have never seen a holistic, undisturbed, normal physiological immediate postpartum period. They are too busy cutting the umbilical cord, separating the baby from its mother, hurriedly performing all sorts of unnecessary procedures so they can move on to the next room to do it all over again. Common practices such as drying, suctioning, immediate vitamin K injections, weighing and measuring, all disrupt the mother/child bond. When the bond is disturbed, it can have long lasting effects on everyone involved.

Many hospitals now advertise that they "allow" skin-to-skin contact, although unfortunately in most settings, the permitted or advertised skin-to-skin contact means for the first few *minutes* after birth, before they take baby away to start doing all the routine procedures. When in fact, skin-to-skin contact should be undisturbed for the first few hours, and then continued over the weeks of the fourth trimester.

Social media recently showed a hospital in America that charged a mum $39.35 for the pleasure of skin-to-skin contact with her baby after birth. Imagine our hospitals making money from women and babies doing what is natural – what is their right: being together. Talk to your hospital about their routine practices and procedures.

Four Important things to know immediately after birth

1. There is no need for the baby to leave your arms.

   Most babies born gently, from healthy mums, come out, take a breath, and blink into the world. Keep in mind "all resources come to baby; not baby to resources": if your PCP wants to check your baby's temperature, listen to his heart rate or lungs, this can all be done on your chest.

   Note: She will only need to be moved if she needs help to start breathing.

2. Routine suctioning of your baby is not needed.

   Babies know how to cough and sneeze and clear their airways. Unless a baby needs help to breathe, she should not be suctioned. Suctioning can affect breastfeeding, because babies are smart; if the first thing in their mouth is painful and rough, they will spit out the next thing – the nipple. (Routine stomach washing is also not supported by research[5.] and is uncomfortable for your baby; decline that, too.)

3. Delayed cord clamping/cutting is essential.

   There is a huge body of evidence supporting the benefits of not cutting the umbilical cord right away, but sadly it is still routine practice by many PCPs.

   The World Health Organisation defines delayed clamping and cutting to be 3–5 minutes after the birth. I would consider this a minimum; it is even better to wait until the pulsations stop (once all the blood has finished transferring from the placenta to the baby – you can feel this yourself by touching the umbilical cord), which can take 10–20 minutes. In an ideal world the cord would not be cut until after the placenta is delivered.

   Benefits include reduced childhood anemia, and better fine motor skills at 4 years of age. Babies need their full blood volume!

   http://archpedi.jamanetwork.com/Mobile/article.aspx?articleid=2296145

4. The benefits of skin-to-skin contact

....

[5.] "Status of gastric lavage in neonates born with meconium stained amniotic fluid: a randomized controlled trial" Lokraj Shah, Gauri Shankar Shah, Rupa Rajbhandari Singh, Hanoon Pokharel, and Om Prakash Mishra. Published online 2015 Oct 31 PMC4628437
https://www.ncbi.nlm.nih.gov/pmc/articles/PMC4628437/

The baby knows the mother's body from the inside, so getting to know her from the outside with undisturbed contact helps ease the huge transition from aquatic life to life on land. The baby's heart rate, temperature and respirations will all regulate with greater ease.

This contact is just as essential for the mother, as it is for her baby. Her chances of postnatal complications like hemorrhage are greatly reduced when baby is kept on her chest rather than taken across the room. Remember, oxytocin is also required *after* the baby is out for the birth of the placenta, and to help the uterus squeeze down on that open placental site.

If your baby is taken out of your arms and taken to the other side of the room, your body will start out on a different physiological process. Separation is not normal; it will start a sympathetic response of fight or flight, which, as we know, blocks those lovely hormones of bonding and attaching.

Birth of the placenta

The placenta is the great life-giver: I would like to do a coffee table book that places photos of placentas beside the food journals of mothers! It fascinates me to see how the quality and integrity of a placenta depends a lot on the type of food the woman has eaten, whether it was mostly processed or mostly fresh.

Placentas are soft and usually weigh around 500 grams. They are very capable of making their way out on their own and are commonly born anywhere from 10 to 30 minutes after the birth of the baby. They are born with the most ease when there is no separation between mother and baby – skin-to-skin contact, and baby nuzzling or sucking at the nipple. This all generates the oxytocin necessary for the surges that help release the placenta.

I ask for birth partners to stay present and available for this part of the process. Once the placenta is born, we can start the birthday party

From Fear To Love

celebration, but not before. Mum still needs to be able to maintain focus and connection with her body; this is an important part of the process.

········

Do

········

- Connect with your baby and your body as it moves down and out of your body

- Ask your PCP about catching your own baby

- Remember birth is not something that happens *to you*; it is something that *you do.*

- Discuss your PCP's routine procedures immediately after birth.

- Remember that unless your baby needs urgent medical care at birth, do everything to avoid her being out of someone's loving arms after birth. She has just literally been through a life or death experience and needs your close, loving reassurance.

- Find out about the benefits of delayed cord clamping.

Note: There are some circumstances when skin-to-skin with mum is not possible, and in these instance, the next best place is-skin to-skin with the second parent or the birth companion.

CHAPTER 20

....

Surgery

"There is no scientific evidence that doing over 10% of births with a Caesarean improves the outcome for the woman or improves the outcome for the baby."
Marsden Wagner MD, author, perinatologist and perinatal epidemiologist

For many women, the biggest fear surrounding birth is the idea of being cut. The World Health Organisation (WHO) says that 10% of women need surgery to birth their babies. Each of us must ask ourselves, "What if I beautifully and lovingly prepare and check every single box on the list and end up with a Caesarean?"

Personally, for my birth, I:

- planned a home birth with a midwife;
- have the water birth tub ready;
- have my full support team in place;
- continually work with my fears;
- consciously work at being relaxed and connected to my breath, my baby and the process; and
- feel *excited* and confident when I thought about myself and my baby's birth.

I know, though, that despite all these preparations I might require a Caesarean. I feel grateful that I don't see a Caesarean as a failure, but I know many women who do feel that way after having one.

Even this big fear can be turned into a big love, we can choose to love a Caesarean surgery, to fully participate in it and accept it as a possible, positive outcome. It might be needed to get our beloved babies safely into our arms. Practice saying this affirmation out loud over the coming months: "A Caesarean can be my positive bridge into motherhood."

Reviewing the process of working with fear guides described in Chapter 8, here are some facts to start with:

- Caesarean birth is birth.

The WHO estimates that, when used appropriately, 10-15 percent of babies need to be born by abdominal surgery. We most likely won't know if we are in that 10% until we are in labor.

- Today, Caesarean births range widely from 1 in every 4 babies, to 1 in every 3, and in some private practices up to 85% of babies are born by Caesarean.

The chances of having a Caesarean depend on what country you live in, whether you are being cared for in a public or a private facility (the rate is higher in private facilities), the type of PCP you are giving birth with (midwife or obstetrician) and your chosen location of birth (home or hospital or hospital to hospital). Many PCPs have a Caesarean rate as low as 2–4%.

Medically indicated caesareans fall into two categories: emergency or planned.

- Emergency Caesareans help mothers and babies who are in distress. The most common indications include lack of blood supply, toxemia, severe high blood pressure, infection of the uterus, or hemorrhage.

- Planned medical Caesareans occur before labor starts, and indications include placenta previa or previous classical Caesarean scar (vertical) or previous uterine surgeries.

Common reasons given for Caesareans today include:

Dilation problems
Auspicious date
Big baby
Small baby
Small pelvis
Fibroids
Cord Around the neck of baby
Failure to progress – labor is too long and slow
Breech position
Twins
IVF
Baby's position
Posterior baby
Fetal Distress
Placenta too near the cervix
Previous caesarean
Baby not engaged
Mum afraid of vaginal birth
Baby passes 'due' date
Failed induction
Doctor leaving on holiday
"Less risky"

This list is longer than ever before in history; I am sure you can add to it, based on what you have heard from your friends, or maybe even experienced.

The good news is that the surgery has become so advanced today, it is considered routine and nothing like the risky procedure our foremothers had to go through. Having said that, it is still major surgery and has more potential risks for mums and babies both in both the short and the long term.

How to avoid a Caesarean

- Choosing a PCP with a low Caesarean rate is the most important factor.

- The location of birth: in all the studies ever done on home vs. hospital birth, home birth always comes out as having fewer Caesarean births. However, location also refers to what hospital you choose, as protocols vary hugely from hospital to hospital. It is your job to find out which ones in your area are the most friendly towards natural birth..

- How you looked after yourself in pregnancy – nutrition, exercise, mental preparedness, relaxation practices you have put in place – will help you to be fit to do the work yourself.

- Understanding the best position for the baby and knowing how to support her to get there can also be vitally important.

- An aligned support team will ensure that you are only required to have a Caesarean when truly indicated.

- Hire a doula

Note: Again, you can check all these boxes and still have a surgical birth; no one of us knows for sure whether it will be our journey. However, these measures will reduce your chances by a large percentage.

My ideal Caesarean birth

You can do a lot to overcome any potential disappointment should it turn out that you need a Caesarean. You can choose to own this procedure right now. See it. Feel it.

Ask yourself:

- Who is with me?

- How do I want to feel?

- What music is playing?

- How will I help my baby understand what will/is/has happened?

- How can I reduce the shock for him/her?

- How can I safeguard his/her experience as much as what is in my control?

- Who is on my team during my recovery period?

A Caesarean contingency plan

This is my contingency plan if I need to have a Caesarean, a plan where I can still have a say and be in the leading role as far as possible.

I discussed them point by point with my PCP. Because my PCP was a midwife and would not have performed surgery, I also needed to have this discussion with my back-up obstetrician and the hospital. I had opened up the discussion with my husband long before that, of course.

Please add to and change this plan to make it yours.

I want labor to begin on its own; I want my baby to pick its birthday.(This is not possible if you have placenta previa, discuss with your PCP)

I will take the time I need to let my body know everything is OK. I will assure my body I have given permission for what is about to happen and that we are in safe hands. I will walk myself to the theatre (unless my condition does not allow), where only the necessary people will be allowed in the room. Everyone in the room will introduce themselves to me before we begin. They will turn the temperature to slightly warmer than usual for me and my baby.

My partner will be in the room with me; he will be just beside me. Feeling his cheek on mine will feel good. I am able to relax, because I trust he knows all of my wishes for the baby and will pre-empt whatever I forget or am physically unable to do.

I will stay psychically connected to my baby while on the table. I will keep myself calm and connected with my breath to help keep my baby relaxed and also to help the surgery go as smoothly as it can.

My baby will hear my voice while it is being born, so it knows it is in the right place. I will reassure baby I am there (If I am unable to, my partner will do the same). I will hear my baby's cry right away, strong and present. I will feel elated, overflowing with joy and relief.

The cord will remain intact and our baby will be passed directly to me. My partner will be the one to discover if we have a boy or girl. I will have skin-to-skin contact on the table. We will prepare for this in advance with the front of my gown open and having a warmed blanket ready for baby. (Note to self: remember to put the emergency space blanket in my hospital bag.)

I will have one arm free, so I can touch my baby. No one will announce the sex of my baby, we are supported to discover that ourselves.

All routine newborn procedures will be delayed and discussed with us first, like giving Vitamin K injection. My baby and partner will be able to stay in recovery with me, and my loving support person and my partner will help me to get our baby to the breast .

I will be kind and gentle with myself in the first few days. I will give my body the time it needs to stay quiet and heal. I will heal quickly, because I am so strong and healthy leading up to surgery.

* * *

I can picture the entire process now, and it doesn't feel too bad. And while I know the circumstances might not allow everything on my list, I trust that my team is aware of my desires and intentions, respects them and will do their best.

The healing process

For yourself

- Give yourself plenty of permission to go slowly

- Know your milk might come in slowly; consider arranging milk donations to have on standby so you don't need to stress it

- It might help to write your story, your feelings, sooner than later while they are still fresh.

- Share your feelings openly.

- If you are angry, let it out – scream into a pillow, punch a pillow, do whatever you need to get an emotional release.

- Hire a postnatal massage woman who can nurture you.

For the baby

- Talk to her about her birth and explain what happened and why. Let her know you were always there waiting for her.

- If she seems angry, that's OK. Let her 'talk'; she needs to share her story too.

- Your baby might like to be swaddled and kept tight when not having skin-to-skin contact.

- No bathing – let's support that microbiome.

- More skin-to-skin contact – with immediate family members if it can't be you; think: relaxing the nervous system, feeling safe and healthy microbiome.

- Consider taking baby for a biodynamic craniosacral session or osteopathy.

....
Do
....

- Make your ideal Caesarean list. Close your eyes and see it all happening. Let some of that fear dissipate, it doesn't need to have power over you.

- Discuss your list with your PCP.

- Include your partner and baby in planning to be Caesarean ready.

- Find out what fears your partner has about Caesarean birth.

- Do whatever you need to do to transform your fear of a Caesarean birth into owning the potential for a love-based, gentle, Caesarean birth for you and your baby.

- Plan for how you will help your body heal, should you need a Caesarean.

A Whole New World

CHAPTER 21

························

The Fourth Trimester

"A newborn baby has only three demands. They are warmth in the arms of its mother, food from her breasts, and security in the knowledge of her presence. Breastfeeding satisfies all three."
Grantly Dick-Read MD/OBGYN, author of *Childbirth Without Fear*

And then, just like that, your little one is in your arms. Well done, Mama!

The transition from preparing *for* something to being *in* something is huge. I was recently having a biodynamic craniosacral (BCST) session with a new mum and while on my table she was sobbing, "I miss being pregnant. I miss being in that expectant stage. It is all over."

We can help ease this huge transition from pregnancy to new motherhood by treating the first month after birth as a fourth trimester. Both mums and babies benefit from taking the first month after birth to nest into a fourth trimester together.

What is a fourth trimester?

Neither mum nor baby is ready to be out and about in the world immediately after birth. You have opened wide physically, emotionally and spiritually to allow the passage of your baby, and babies need time to adapt to living on land. Babies want to be brought slowly into this big world of stimulus and activity, and your body wants time to heal; they are both open and vulnerable.

It is not only your baby who has been born; you have also been born as a mother.

The slowing down you did during pregnancy, and especially during the third trimester, has prepared you to slow down even further now. Forget that to-do list. This is time to let go even more of the pressure you put on yourself. Instead, shower yourself with self-love, kindness and gentleness. This is a whole new world, a whole new reality. Please give yourself permission to relax into *being*.

> "The world stands still for while – let it. Your new baby doesn't need much at all. Just you.. You, you, you. And swaddling."
> Kyra, first baby, America/Singapore

The fourth trimester is also an important time for dads/other parent to connect and get to know baby. Ideally, they will have arranged their work schedule so they can stay home for the first two weeks, to nurture you and get to know and help care for baby. It is a great way to establish the family bond. Dads shouldn't be left out of this juicy time!

There are many beautiful, postnatal traditions around the world, some that I have been lucky to participate in, that honor the motherbaby dyad (the term used to acknowledge you both as an inseparable unit). The tradition of nurturing the nurturer is a beautiful tradition: daily massages and warm baths, belly wraps, warm breast milk-supportive foods – in some places this continues for 28 to 40 days after birth.

> "I prepared for the first month by letting everyone know that I wouldn't be leaving home for 40 days. To bond with baby, to learn breastfeeding and to recover with very little stimulus. Fortunately, I lived in a place where I had full-time house help and I also had a massage every day for 40 days to help me recover physically, and my mom with me for emotional support."
> Tonia, first and second baby, Canada/India

Western culture is the opposite, and the expectation and pressure to 'bounce back' right after giving birth is huge. I am here to encourage you to forget what society expects of you and get cozy.

Keep in mind, if the choir didn't sing from somewhere above when your baby was placed on your chest, or if you didn't feel that overwhelming sense of love that women talk about, don't worry – that is also normal. Not every love is love at first sight. Some love needs time to grow. Think of this as your babymoon time.

> "My cousin told me that she read that not everyone falls in love with their baby right away. That was so important as I didn't fall in love with my son when he was born. I loved him but didn't have an immediate bond."
>
> Mary-Signe first baby, USA/India

For baby

Human mammals are born premature; we are very different from all the other mammals who can walk and follow their mothers around minutes after birth.

The reason is that we have big brains; our large neocortex doesn't have the luxury of growing *inside* the mother for as long as it needs to; birth wouldn't work if we gestated for the additional months we would need to be ready for the world. Instead, our babies come early and have to trust that they won't be left behind.

When you imagine what your baby needs in the first month after birth, think of a baby kangaroo, a joey: low stimulation, loads of skin-to-skin contact, warm and snug. I often get calls from nervous mums in the middle of the night. "My baby won't stop crying; his crying is loud and intense, and I think he is in pain. Do I need to go to the emergency room?"

I always ask what happened during the day. What was the activity level, how many visitors came by? In 95% of those phone calls I get the answer: "Well, we took the bus to have lunch with a friend, then we taxied to the mall to pick up a few things I needed for baby." Or "We had a constant stream of visitors today, and baby was passed around a lot. It felt exhausting."

Your baby's nervous system isn't ready for all that stimulation. They usually respond in one of two ways:

- shutting down and sleeping a lot; or

- not being able to shut down and instead letting the frustration and stimulation out of their little systems by crying and screaming until they shut down from exhaustion.

For Mum

After a gentle birth, most women feel great, like a superhuman who can conquer the world. For those first three days, you have adrenaline and feel-good hormones playing interchangeably. You might not sleep much because you are too excited, admiring the beauty you have created.

Recently, a home birth mum who came for BCST told me that she had had a doctor attending her home birth and very little home care follow-up after the birth; she was shattered. "I felt so good in the first 24 hours after birth that on the second morning, I got up and cleaned the house from top to bottom. I felt so energized." She then recounted how she had spent the next four days in bed feeling like she had been run over by a truck. She had used the energy boost her body gave her for sleepless nights – for the wrong purpose.

"Your body is tired (and sore). I felt the rush and energy I had from the pregnancy hormones leave my body for a few days – this was tough, as I loved how they made me feel. These first few weeks are so precious with your little one – and you can just see that they want to be kept safe, and warm and close to you. Try keep this time sacred."
Melissa, first baby, South Africa/Singapore

This is a potential problem with home birth. It is too easy to get up, wander off to your kitchen and start making something to eat, forgetting that something huge just happened to your body.

CASE STUDY

I was attending a home birth last year. The mum had an incredibly inspiring birth –she was a lion roaring her baby into her hands in the water. Then she rested and marvelled, got out of the tub, gently pulled out her own placenta, sat down and started nursing. She amazed me, as all women at birth do, but I was even more enchanted than usual because she had conceived her baby with IVF. As I felt my own IVF journey approaching, I was so inspired by how she reclaimed what started out as a medical process into something that she owned and exalted in. (She later turned into one of my IVF big sisters. She had my back, was holding my intentions with me and was cheering me along. I am so grateful to have seen multiple, full-power IVF babies born at home since then.)

This roaring mamma felt great! Two hours after the birth, I was in the other room doing my charting and drinking a cup of tea, and I turned around and much to my horror saw mamma *carrying* her 2-year-old on her hip to the toilet. It felt normal to her to do that.

Remember: Respecting your body during the fourth trimester is the primary act of self-love. Your organs are all moving and finding their way back to their usual location, you will start to producing milk, have a healing placenta site, and emotions that are going to start going up and down.

> **Note:** This simple saying is a good guide: after birth spend five days in the bed, five days on the bed, five days around the bed.

> "Rest up (ideally in bed). Give your body the time and calm environment to recover. [It] has done a great job! Don't have visitors. They can come to see baby later. This is about you and your new little family. Spend as much quality time with your baby as possible, and cuddle it as much as you can. Time passes too fast, and baby grows too quickly."
> Anonymous, second baby, Singapore

I promise you, no matter how hard it is to stay quiet, the physically quieter you are in the first days, weeks and even month, the better you will feel at four weeks, at three months, at six months after the birth.

Creating the scene

Plan for your fourth trimester well in advance. As much as possible, all household responsibilities like preparing meals, cleaning and other household chores should be delegated for the first few weeks. To make this happen, who will you need on your team?

Get creative and consider your birth partner, friends, family, postnatal doulas or hired help. Cook up healthy meals to freeze in your last few weeks of pregnancy.

An ideal scenario is that your primary responsibility during this period (as a minimum, the first two weeks) is to learn to breastfeed, get to know your little one and let your body rest. Tell all your friends that you will let them know when you are ready to introduce your baby. If they want to help/see you, ask them to bring a meal or come and spend 20 minutes doing some light housework.

Create a little nest in your bedroom so you have everything you need within reach. Nappy-changing, eating – everything can happen inside your little nest to begin with.

Note: Babies don't require a ton of stuff, avoid overwhelming yourself to all sorts of plastics and things to put baby down in. On Love Based Birth you will find a list of must have's to gather as you prepare for baby.

"Living in Singapore, I had heard about the 'confinement' that many Asian mothers do after giving birth. I loved this idea but chose to call it instead a 'hibernation'. I insisted to my partner, friends, family and community, that I wanted 40 days of hibernation with no visitors, no work, no appointments, etc. As it turned out, my beloved really helped to create this cocoon so that I had hardly any visitors and could hibernate with Baby as much as possible. One of my friends arranged for meals to be delivered for a week; I had other friends on hand to deliver items from markets/grocery stores; and my husband took time off his freelancing work to look after the home, laundry, food, birth registration appointments, everything! I also had 10 days of belly wraps from a dear Malaysian friend, which helped me healing so much. Essentially, we created an environment where I could be braless, in pyjamas, massaged and nourished, and totally free as I learned how to breastfeed, to love and nourish our new baby, to heal my body and to fall in love with my husband again as a triad."
Amber, first baby, USA/Singapore

For the dad/other parent

The primary care giver for baby in the fourth trimester is the person who is breastfeeding. Your role as primary supporter is key during this special time. Your main role is to nurture and love your beautiful partner so she has the stamina to nurture and love your little one. While breastfeeding is completely normal, it can take some learning on both mum and baby's side. Your loving gentle presence, reassurance, and encouragement are essential in the learning days.

Sometimes you might feel jealous of the fact that she is the primary person for baby, and that's OK. It is normal. Sometimes you will also feel relieved she is, and that is normal too!

You will also feel overwhelmed and tired; having a new baby is a huge transition for you, too. Remember that on top of that your partner has dramatically shifting hormones, sore nipples, and a body that is recovery from pushing a human out into the world or possibly major abdominal surgery. I would recommend avoiding sentences like: "I don't think you're doing it right," or "She's crying because she is hungry!", especially if she has just been nursing at the breast for the last hour.

Many parents ask me when they can introduce the bottle so dad can have a turn feeding, because he wants to feel close to baby, too, by nurturing her with food.

Here's the thing: daddy, you were not born with breasts that produce milk. It is a job you were simply not made to do. Please let go of the idea that the only way you can bond with your little one is by feeding her.

> "Breastfeeding should not be attempted by fathers with hairy chests, since they can make baby sneeze and give it wind."
> Mike Harding, *The Armchair Anarchist's Almanac*

Introducing a bottle can be very confusing for a little one at this stage because the mechanical rhythm for sucking and swallowing is very different with each process. Drinking from the breast goes something like: suck, suck, suck, suck, let down, swallow, swallow, gulp, swallow, suck, swallow, suck, suck, swallow. And from a bottle it is more like: suck, swallow, suck, swallow, suck, swallow.

These are other ways that you directly nurture and love your baby: do all the nappy changing, massaging, bathing, walking, cuddling, learning to settle her down and having lots of skin-to-skin contact. There have been tons of studies about the benefits of skin to skin contact with dad:

> "The infants in the skin-to-skin group were comforted, that is, they stopped crying, became calmer, and reached a drowsy state earlier than the infants in the cot group. The father can facilitate the development of the infant's pre-feeding behavior in this important period of the newborn infant's life and should thus be regarded as the primary caregiver for the infant during the separation of mother and baby."[6]

Do

- Be gentle and loving with yourself – this is a huge change!

- Co-sleep: have your baby either in your bed or in its own space attached to the bed so you can roll over to breastfeed. Whether you choose to continue to co-sleep after the fourth trimester is not something you need to decide now.

- Allow your baby to teach you.

[6] "Skin-to-skin care with the father after Caesarean birth and its effect on newborn crying and prefeeding behaviour" Erlandsson K1, Dsilna A, Fagerberg I, Christensson K. 2007 Jun;34(2):105-14 PMID:17542814
https://www.ncbi.nlm.nih.gov/pubmed/17542814

- Speak up and don't allow yourself to be bullied by family/ confinement nurses or anyone else on matters of raising your baby.

- Allow your maternal/paternal instinct to rise; put the books down.

- Spend as much time skin-to-skin as you can in the first weeks – baby wants to feel your body and be on your skin. Remember, touch is nutrition. Skin-to-skin also means with the other parent. (Many studies are available documenting the benefits of continued skin-to-skin contact, for example: baby will cry less, breastfeeding will be better established and the new mother's stress levels will also be reduced.)

- Move slowly and respectfully with your body

- Hire someone to come and massage you in the first weeks

- Delegate.

- Take time for sitz baths.

- Talk *to* your baby, not just *about* your baby.

- Remember that your baby is a fully conscious being and can sense what you are feeling, but he probably hasn't figured out yet that he is not part of your body.

- Acknowledge that he hears and feels everything you say about him.

- Talk with your baby about all the things you are doing. When you are working on your latch say, "Open your mouth a little wider so you can get your milk easier. That's it. . We are learning together."

- Give yourself permission to stay in bed in your pajamas.

- Give yourself permission to cry and not get it right all the time.

- Remember that your baby is not trying to manipulate you; it's just that his every single need has to be met by you.

- Have water beside you whenever you are breastfeeding.

- Give yourself permission to take breaks. Hand your baby over to someone else on the team and give yourself some time for you.

- Hold him close. Swaddle him.

- Keep him nice and cozy; it was 37 degrees in your body.

- Forget about schedules and timings.

- Know your baby doesn't want perfection; it wants *you* just as you are.

- Limit visitors – very few to none in the first week, slowly allowing for more in the second if you are ready.

- Lean on your support people; talk on the phone to a friend if you need some perspective.

- I don't usually like lists of don'ts, but here is one:

Don't

- Worry if you feel you have no idea what she wants. That's normal.

- Forget to include your baby in your conversations.

- Put her to sleep down the hall or in another room.

- Let her cry for no reason. If she is crying and you're trying to change his diaper, then pick her up in the middle of the change and tell her you are there and help her to relax.

- Put mittens on her. She needs tactile sense. Those marks on her face from scratching will go away.

- Use soap or other products on her until at least after the first six weeks.

- Take him out to malls and other crowded, stimulating places.

- Only lie her on her back. She needs pressure on all sides of her soft head. During the day when you are awake, let her nap on her side and alternate. A rolled towel behind her works very well for the support she needs to stay on her side.

Dos for dads/other parents

- Attend a breastfeeding class together during pregnancy; this will give you a better idea of ways to support mum and what to expect.

- Make sure mum always has water nearby when breastfeeding.

- Give your baby skin-to-skin contact time with you.

- Do as much of the burping as possible – give her arms a break.

- Become a diaper-changing, burping, swaddling expert.

- Give mum breaks: walk, sway, coo and sing to baby.

- Take the lead on making sure baby gets twice daily sunbaths in the first weeks (see Chapter 24 for how your baby can take safe sunbaths).

- If you are comfortable, take the lead on bathing and massaging.

- Take the lead in household chores, preparing food and buying groceries.

CHAPTER 22

Intuition– Responding To Your Baby's Needs

"Connection is why we're here. We are hardwired to connect with others, it's what gives purpose and meaning to our lives, and without it there is suffering."
Brene Brown, *Daring Greatly*

New parenthood is a confusing place today; there are so many opinions and so many books all giving conflicting advice: co-sleep, create a nursery, breastfeed on demand, schedule feeding, pick baby up when it cries, don't pick baby up – it goes on and on.

One of the popular methods is based on scheduling, controlling and separating, rather than responding to your baby's needs. How horrible! Yet it has been picked up and become the guide for hundreds of thousands of new parents.

Is the approach of following our PCPs blindly during pregnancy and surrendering the decision-making process to them affecting our abilities as new parents? Are we so used to someone else deciding things for us that we feel it is easier to leave it to other individuals and organizations to decide for us how we want to parent?

Again, it is easy to again let the fear creep in and dictate our decision-making process:

- "Don't put your baby in your bed, it will never leave."

- "Don't hold your baby all the time, you will spoil her."

- "Don't pick him up when he cries; he is just trying to control you."

What would new parenting look like if instead we allowed our intuition to lead us?

Intuition

Let your intuition be your guide in all the decisions you make. My experience is that women who have the toughest time of the new motherhood period do so because they are forcing themselves to someone else's beliefs or expectations, not their own.

Allow your infinite self to teach you things that you won't find in books.

> "As a first-time mum, I was so worried about doing things right that I didn't listen to my mummy intuition as much as I needed to; I was too scared. After visiting with my sister in the US and realizing that I was just putting too much pressure on myself, I relaxed a lot more, read less books and tried to just do what was best for me and my baby. The second time around, I was much more connected to my intuition. I listened less to everyone's advice and just did what I felt was right for my baby and me. I think being connected to your intuition is so important and key to getting through the tough times without beating yourself up."
> Dao, second baby, Singapore

The slowing down you did during pregnancy, and especially during the third trimester, will serve you well during this period. All that time you spent quieting yourself so you could hear your intuitive whisper – that was in preparation for these sleep-deprived moments.

This is another incredible opportunity to see deeply inside yourself; those old friends "unworthy" and "not good enough" and feelings of guilt and shame might pay frequent visits, and that's OK too. Acknowledge them, then find your way back to your breath and create a new affirmation. You might feel more vulnerable than ever before, ecstatic one minute and sad the next. It won't be easy, and it's not meant to be. You are normal. New motherhood is a bumpy ride, and the better you feel about yourself, your birth, and the choices you made, the better you will be able to bounce along that road without falling off your seat.

Try to remember this is a moment in time; before you know it, everything will change again.

Baby's intuition

Babies are incredibly intuitive characters too – after all, our intuition sits outside the cognitive, rationalizing brain and inside the sensing, feeling brain. They do not over-think things like we do. They simply express whatever their feeling states are.

Babies exploring through touch to learn about their environments – getting to know every corner of the placenta, their umbilical cords, their own bodies. Sucking their fingers, their thumbs, rubbing their noses, scratching their ears: it was so much easier for them to access their hands in the shrinking apartment of the uterus than it is out here. While feeling a belly in a prenatal appointment this week I was wiggling a little head back and forth, and there was the familiar outline of a little hand: it felt like I had caught the baby in mid ear-scratch.

For your baby breastfeeding, which we'll look at in the next chapter, is all about touch. Thousands of messages get delivered to their brains via the nerve receptors at the end of their little fingers – there are 2500 nerve receptors per square centimeter in the human hand. They want to feel the breast and even knead the breast. Have you watched kittens suckle?

When we put gloves on babies, we disturb their learning, we interfere with their ability to rely on their intuitive sense. Have you ever tried to dial your cell phone in the winter with gloves on? The phone and the touch receptors – it just doesn't work out.

I understand that parents use gloves to prevent the baby scratching its face with those sharp nails and to keep them warm. Look for alternatives to keep them warm, like skin-to-skin contact, and clip their nails while they sleep so they don't scratch their faces.

Keep your baby's hands free to discover their new environments and follow their intuitive sense.

Affirmations for new motherhood

As always, pick two or three that resonate with you and use them on repeat throughout the day.

- Being a good mother takes courage, and today I'm feeling brave.
- I feel safe to show my vulnerability.
- The decisions made by other mothers do not need to dictate mine.
- I am the perfect mother for my baby.
- Fear is only a feeling; it won't hold me back.
- My inner voice guides me in every moment.
- Today I am willing to accept my imperfections.
- Today I choose to love and accept myself.
- I have the strength to take care of all my baby's needs.
- I am a wonderful and capable mother.
- Mothering is easier when I let go of trying to control every detail.
- My mother's intuition leads me in the right direction.

> "I have always been intuitive, but the whole process from pregnancy to birth has added another level of understanding and trusting my own instincts when it comes to my baby."
> Tanishq, first baby, Singapore

- I love taking good care of myself and my baby.
- I give myself permission to ask for help
- I give myself permission to stay in bed and rest.
- I love myself.

Do

- Listen for and trust your intuition.
- Plan ahead.
- Be gentle with yourself.
- Cancel everything on your calendar for at least two weeks, and ideally four.
- Try using affirmations when you are feeling low or in a storm.

CHAPTER 23

Breastfeeding And The First Three Days

"A baby nursing at a mother's breast is an undeniable
affirmation of our rootedness in nature."
David Suzuki, scientist, environmental activist

Breasting is simple and normal, but it is not always easy. Having a good understanding of how to get a good latch for baby, positions to try, ways to trouble-shoot problems like engorgement and sore nipples, before birth, will go a long way to support you in the moment.

The more support you get in the early days, the better chance you have of breastfeeding for longer. The current recommendation is to breastfeed until 12 months of age.

Preparing for breastfeeding

Take a breastfeeding class. Ideally your primary partner will also attend the class with you so he/she knows how to get involved and takes a supporting role. Build your support team. Find out who the postnatal doulas, midwives, lactation consultants or breastfeeding counsellors are in your area who do home visits.

I am a big fan of mothers learning to hand-express milk during the last few weeks of pregnancy. It is an important skill to have, because if for any reason your baby cannot suckle (for example, he needs to go to the NICU), you will be able to extract those drops of liquid gold your body is producing and hand-feed your baby. If your breasts become very engorged (full) when your milk comes in, you will be glad that you know how to that hand-express.

Own this part. Get to know your breasts. There are some good videos on the Love Based Birth website on how to hand-express milk. If you have flat or inverted nipples or suspect any other reason that breastfeeding might be challenging for you at the start, you might want to store up a bit of colostrum. It is a substance that just keeps replenishing itself, so you don't have to worry that it will be used up.

Colostrum = liquid gold

The wondrous colostrum is already in your breasts during pregnancy, patiently waiting for baby by the end of the third trimester. You might see it if you give your breast a squeeze, or you might see it even if you don't. Just know that it is there, waiting, a silent, magical superfood. It is affectionately referred to as "liquid gold" because it is full of antibodies and immunoglobulins to help boost your baby's immune system. It is the perfect stomach coating for a gut system that is still underdeveloped and "sieve-like". It also has a laxative affect and helps your little one with their first poos.

Milk commonly comes in on the third day, so for the first three days, the baby will be drinking colostrum. There won't be vast quantities, which is why your baby will want to come to the breast very frequently. I recommend using both breasts per feeding while baby is drinking colostrum to help support your milk coming in. That means if after 15 minutes baby is still drinking at the breast, you can switch her to the other breast to continue drinking. If your nipples are sore use one breast at a time.

General guidelines

The first 24 hours

Don't worry about matching any rhythms during the first 24 hours of your baby's life you can both rest. Babies are tired after birth, too! Just offer your breast to your baby whenever he first wakes up.

- Disturb baby as little as possible.
- She will like to be swaddled when not having skin-to-skin contact.
- No need to wake her up for feeds – let her rest and recover from the birth.
- Check she is not cold – feel her hands and nose.
- When she wakes, offer the breast first.
- Limit visitors.
- Get as much rest as you can to recover from the birth, as the next few days will be busy – nap and rest whenever she does.
- Do not bath her.
- Baby stays in the room with you.
- Put a little coconut oil on her bottom for ease of cleaning meconium poo.
- Using both breasts with colostrum per feed is OK.
- If this is your second or third baby or more and the after cramps are intense while breastfeeding you can take acetaminophen (paracetamol) as needed. Try herbs like cramp root bark.

Day 2

After the first 24 hours of rest, your baby will need to drink from your breast every 2– 3 hours in the day and every 3–4 at night.

It is common to need to wake a baby up to feed. He is used to constant placenta nutrition and may not recognize a grumbling belly as a sign to wake up and tell you he is hungry. This is a learned response; he will learn quickly but needs you to manage it for him at the beginning.

Other babies might wake more frequently than 2-3 hours to ask for the breast, and this is normal too. Those frequent feeds help the milk to come in and protect babies against jaundice.

- Your baby might suckle a lot or might want to sleep a lot.

- Follow your intuition and his lead (unless that is a very sleepy lead).

- If there are any blood spots or specific areas to clean on baby you can gentle wash them off with a warm cloth. If you had a water birth and your baby is clean, there is no need.

Note: Try to keep as much amniotic fluid on him as possible so he can still have that familiar smell in his vastly changed world – no big washes or submerging baths today.

- The second night can be busy: your baby might be cranky, missing his cozy water world. Nap during the day whenever he sleeps and continuing to keep visitors to a minimum will help.

- Get in the habit today of offering baby to burp either over your shoulder or sitting draped forward over your hand. Offer burps:

  – to wake him up when he sleeps in the middle of feeding

  – after feeding

  – between feeds

- Start sunbaths today. Hopefully you have natural light in your postnatal room if you are in hospital, or at home, please don't sit in the dark with all the curtains closed. Letting in light will help your little one to deal with the changes happening in his body, like ridding itself of extra red blood cells.

- Start your sitz baths if you are already at home.

Day 3: milk day

Day 3 is milk day for many women, but not all. You might have your own way with this like with everything else. Factors surrounding the birth can also affect when your milk comes in, for example, whether you were induced, had increased bleeding after birth, or had a Caesarean.

The milk commonly comes in with a bang! Your body doesn't know if it had twins or triplets and wants to be ready to feed everybody. Your boobs might be hard and sore. This will change as your body figures out supply and demand, but it will take a few days.

Midwives often say, "When the milk flows, so do the tears." If you feel extra teary today, don't worry. That is normal. All those wonderful hormones that made you sick at the beginning of pregnancy, but that you got used to, have left your system. Tears and being extra sensitive often take their place.

> " [I am proudest] that I managed to breastfeed him until now (two years) even after all our challenges at the start! After birth, I didn't have much milk, and to make matters worse I didn't get to have skinto-skin as he was transferred to NICU due to his lungs having meconium. He was there for ten days, and every day I gave him syringes of my milk. When we reunited, thank God, he latched on like a pro and since then, he's been loving my milk!"
> Ikin, first baby, Singapore

You might also be going home today if you birthed in a hospital, but you don't need to worry because you have already set your support structure in place for once you're home.

Continue as for day 2, with some extra guidance:

- Go extra slowly and gently with yourself; your body is doing big things.

- A low-grade fever (100.3) is considered normal and a sign the milk is on the way.

- A midwife, postnatal doula, lactation supporter can all make the transition to home so much easier.

- Give way to tears and feelings of being overwhelmed if they come; it is normal.

- Ideally, only feed your baby from one breast at each feed (if your milk is in), while your milk is regulating (think overstimulation).

- Manage engorgement if it occurs.

- Take naps when your baby sleeps.

- Stay in bed.

- Producing milk burns many calories – you need more calories for breastfeeding than during pregnancy, so remember to care for yourself with good nurturing foods.

Engorgement

The best thing for engorgement is rest. Milk production is partly why you are staying quiet and in your pajamas while your body is adjusting to this new job.

Some things that can help with engorgement:

- rest;

- alternating warm and cold compresses;

- warm showers and hand-expressing the pressure off;

- feeding frequently; and

- while your baby is nursing, gently massaging that same breast, making sure to work down any chickpea-sized lumps you find

Please don't pump and store milk during this period if your baby is with you and able to latch. You will make the body think it is required to produce that much and engorgement can continue longer.

Remember, this is just a moment in time. By the end of the week things will be different again and getting a little easier. This is the really hard part for many women; you are not alone.

> **Note:** Be sure to call your PCP if you have a fever above 100.3, cannot latch baby to the breast, or develop any red sore spots on your breast.

How do you know baby is hungry?

A cry is a late sign of hunger. Ideally you can catch the early signs that your baby is ready to eat because it will be much easier to latch him in this state than when he is all worked up. A good general standard operating procedure is to offer him a feed as soon as he wakes up and starts to squirm. He will also start to give signals like opening his mouth like a little bird looking for a worm, and suck on his fingers.

Establishing breastfeeding

Breastfeeding positions

Cross-cradle, football, side-lying, laid back – do you know what all this means?

Here is your checklist for a successful feed:

✓ Always bring the baby to the breast, not the breast to the baby.

✓ Pull your baby in close.

✓ Make sure you are both well supported – use props.

✓ Position yourselves tummy to tummy, *not* with your baby's head turned.

✓ Your baby should have her mouth just below your nipple.

✓ Make sure you can see her neck: it should be nice and open; her chin should not be collapsing on her chest.

Cracked nipples

Developing cracks or blisters on your nipples is a sign that your baby in not latched well. It is important to seek out support right away to help correct the latch.

In the meantime, short-term solutions can include:

- air: letting nipples dry

- milk: covering the nipples with breastmilk to help them heal (remember, breastmilk is world's best natural first aid)

- lanolin: a good salve to have on standby

Breastfeeding visualizations

Once you get your baby latched and you are in a comfortable position, find your breath and, just like you did so many times during pregnancy, scan your body and notice where you are holding tension. Breathe into that area to help it relax. Relax your face, your shoulders, your hands and your feet. Notice where everything is relaxing and soften into those areas even more deeply.

- Feel your entire body as a loose, open and receptive vessel; feel rivers of milk flowing from your nipples, not too fast but at just the right pace for your baby.

- Feel a bubble of love and peace all around you and your baby.

- Relax your jaw; smile.

Breastfeeding affirmations

- I am making an abundance of milk for my baby.
- I am good at breastfeeding.
- Frequent nursing is normal.
- My milk flows at the perfect rate for my baby.
- I have unlimited patience with myself and my baby.
- I ask for help and allow others to help me.
- I am grateful for the wisdom of my body.
- I am a strong and loving mother.
- My milk supplies my baby with all the nutrients she needs.
- My baby is gaining weight every day.
- My baby and I enjoy nursing together.
- I can master anything if I do it enough times.
- Babies cry and that is normal; it is not a reflection of anything I am doing wrong.
- I treat myself with kindness and respect.
- Everyday breastfeeding is a little bit easier.

Do

- Breastfeed in the first hour after birth.
- Offer the breast frequently in the first days – frequent feeds help bring the milk.
- Take time to get yourself in a comfortable positon; use props

- Do your best to find positions where your wrist can be relaxed

- Bring baby to the breast, don't lean down to bring your breast to baby

- Avoid topping up baby with formula, glucose water, or anything else, unless you have a special circumstance you are working with

- Consider having a bag of a friend's breastmilk in the fridge, just in case you need it.

- Be gentle with yourself

- Feed both breasts in the first days when producing colostrum.

- Feed one breast at a time once the milk is in.

- Don't use a breast pump unless baby is not with you or cannot latch.

- Make sure your bra is not too tight (no underwire!) and causing creases anywhere; this will encourage breast infection.

- Avoid introducing a pacifier for at least the first month.

- Eat well – your body is burning a lot of calories.

- Hand-express if your nipple is too hard for your baby to latch onto.

- Get plenty of rest – milk production is a big job.

- Wait until six months to start any foods with your baby.

- Use affirmations.

CHAPTER 24

Newborn Care

"I have been with you, from the beginning of time".
Rumi

The desire for a gentle birth flows naturally into gentle baby care. As with everything, there are different ideas about what gentle baby care looks like. In this chapter, I'll share my top points to consider.

Products

One of the aspects of gentle parenting includes being mindful of the products you use on or near babies' skins.

Their skin is very sensitive and interacts with everything it meets. It is common in the first days and weeks to see rashes, red spots and even acne. A lot of this is normal and caused by their pores opening and getting used to dust, fabrics, sweat and everything else that is a part of land living. The fewer irritants they encounter, the better. This is why I suggest you to evaluate the products you use in your house before the birth.

You should use a natural detergent on all her bedding and clothes, and on your clothes, and in fact on those of any primary care giver, so you may as well switch over your entire household. Be aware of perfumes, as well. Babies spend a lot of time up by your neck for burping and settling, and you don't want their faces and little noses to be buried in your favorite cologne.

She doesn't need soaps, shampoos, powders or lotions. Many of the brands that advertise themselves as 'newborn skin friendly', 'baby safe' or 'hypoallergenic' can have a long list of ingredients including harmful chemicals. Get used to reading labels, and don't use anything with names you can't pronounce.

There are a thousand gentle baby product lines on the market. Some of the good natural ingredients include calendula, chamomile and lanolin. However, I would save the fortune you could spend in that direction and instead only use coconut oil for skin care. Because it is antifungal, antibacterial and moisturizing, it is perfect for their sensitive skin. They don't have hormones, so they don't smell if they sweat. They are on a breast milk diet, and are not out playing in the mud. Coconut oil and a good bum cream in case of nappy rash should do it.

In the 1980s, the 'back to sleep' campaign began as a prevention for Sudden Infant Death Syndrome, and at that time the belief was that the babies' sleeping position was causing the deaths. Some researchers suggest that the position itself is not the reason for the deaths, but rather the gasses coming off the chemicals in mattresses[7].

Investing in a natural mattress for your bed during pregnancy is a very wise health investment. If your baby is in a co-sleeper or cot beside your bed, please also make sure its mattress is chemical free.

Diapers and global waste

We each have a responsibility to look after this beautiful planet we inhabit, and we need to know how bad disposable diapers are for the earth. Because of their plastic and chemical composition, it takes each diaper roughly 500 years to decompose. In many countries, diapers

....

[7] Sprott TJ. The Cot Death Cover-up? Auckland: Penguin Environmental-NZ, 1996. Richardson BA. Sudden infant death syndrome: A possible primary cause. Jour Forensic Science Society 1994;34:199-204.

are ending up at the bottom of the sea and otherwise in landfill. Each child produces about one ton of landfill waste every year he wears a Huggy or a Pamper. If using disposable choose an eco-friendly one.

When deciding on diapering, it doesn't have to be fully cloth or fully disposable – you can find a middle ground that works for your family.

These are my gentle diapering guidelines:

- For the first few days, disposables might be easier because of the meconium –the first poo they make, which is like black tar: it is a stain that is nearly impossible to clean out of cloth diapers.

- Try to buy a diaper that is eco-friendly and made by a responsible company.

- Babies are born without hip sockets, so take care to lift both legs at a time rather than just one leg, or get used to gently turning her from side to side when getting a diaper on and off. (There is a demonstration video on the Love Based Birth website).

- Strange colors: if you see a little red or orange in the diaper during the first week, don't panic. Little girls get almost like a little period – it's from your hormones and is normal. Little boys can have an orange discharge as their livers cleanse out the excess cells.

- Girls will have thick, white discharge, and that is normal. There is no need to clean up inside the vagina of little girls; wipe it externally and the rest will come when it is ready. Always wipe front to back.

- With boys, it is no longer recommended that you to retract the penis while cleaning; it will retract on its own when it is ready. Try to point his penis down when you close the diaper, otherwise he can pee up and out of his diaper and onto his cord stump or face.

- Fold the top of the diaper down so the cord can breathe and dry.

Nappy wipes

Even the wipes that claim to be organic or natural usually contain chemicals; get the best you can find and reserve them for using when you are out. If you need a nesting project at the end of the third trimester you can find recipes online (including on Love Based Birth) for making your own.

At home, the best way to wash baby's bottom is with plain water. Until the cord stump falls off, you can use small baby wash cloths and a bowl of warm water. You can start a color-coded system, for example, colored washcloths are for the bottom and white cloths are for the face and rest of the body.

Once the cord stump has fallen off and you have more confidence in handling your baby, the easiest way to clean the bottom is by rinsing it under the sink tap.

Cord care

Forget those antiseptic sprays and ointments you have been sent home from the hospital with. In my entire career as I midwife I don't remember seeing a single cord infection. Alcohols and other antiseptics are very drying and harsh on sensitive skin and have a very strong odor for baby.

Natural cord care includes:

- delaying the first submerging bath until it falls off : this will prevent it getting moist and further delaying the healing process;

- folding the diaper down below it, so it can get plenty of air;

- using a clean cloth dipped in warm clean water to wipe away any oozy, yellow or green pus-y bits;

- keeping an eye on it to ensure it does not develop a funky smell or redness on the surrounding the skin, and if it does, checking with your midwife.

Swaddling

Babies usually like to be cozy and tight in the first few weeks after birth: everything they know is soft and tight and warm. A large percentage of crying/anxiety from babies on my house visits is in part resolved with just getting them a bit cozier. Often the house is too cold for how they are dressed, or they are feeling too much space around them and want to be swaddled.

When swaddling:

- Let your baby's hips stay mobile; don't 'cinch up' the legs when tying the swaddle.

- Try a hands-free swaddle; your baby will like to be able to put her hands near her face.

- Babies need to use their muscles, too, so don't keep them in a swaddle all day.

Sleeping

When mothers follow their instinct rather than their fears or someone else's opinion, their baby will always sleep near where they sleep. Not down the hall – you want to be able to hear them, to check on them without having to get out of bed and leave your bedroom to find them. This is exhausting, because waking up frequently in the early days to check if they are still breathing is normal. Just like baby, you are also used to them being a constant part of you, not separate, so it might feel strange to start with. Having them always within arm's reach will make this transition easier.

Assuming no drugs or alcohol have been consumed, you can trust you will awake with every groan and grunt your baby makes. Your instincts are on high alert.

> "Intuition connects us with our babies, I always find it funny to wake up seconds before the cry comes from my little one."
> Aurore, second baby, VBAC France/Singapore

Mums ask me a lot, "My baby sounds like a truck driver/little piggy/old man when she's sleeping. Is it normal for her to be so loud?" It is.

If you still feel too nervous about having your baby in your bed, then co-sleepers that hook onto the side of your bed, or sit a little higher on your bed like a Cocoonababy; will likely make you feel more confident.

Crying

Babies have all sorts of feelings and stories they want to share with you. One of the ways they do that is by crying. Sometimes your baby will cry even after you have gone through the checklist of:

- feeding
- changing
- burping
- too warm/hot
- needing a cuddle

Do your best to turn on your intuition. What does the cry sound like? What does he need right now? Is she frightened or angry? I read somewhere once that nothing raises the adult blood pressure faster than the sound of a newborn crying. Incredible biology – it means it is impossible to ignore that shriek for help! But if you have absolutely no idea what the cry means, that is OK, too. It's normal not to know sometimes. You won't always know. You're still a wonderful mother. The perfect mother for this little one. She chose *you*. The most important thing is that you are there. Tell her you are there and doing your best, but you don't know what is happening for her.

> "With the first child, I had to learn first to really listen to my intuition. It's there, but I didn't trust myself. Still rather asked others for advice. By the third child, I knew to follow my instincts only. Same for everyday challenges, I know listen to my inner voice in matters around education and raising the kids."
>
> Bea, third baby, German/Singapore

Babies love to be validated. Try sentences along the lines of, "I see you are having a really hard time." Or, "Whatever you are experiencing looks incredibly painful." These will help them to feel that they are heard, and their experiences and feelings are important. I am not a fan of "shushing", because it feels like the exact opposite of validating.

If you are alone with your baby, feeling overwhelmed, she won't stop crying, and you are desperate for a break, do this:

1. Tell her you are at the end of your rope and need to step away for a moment.

2. Put her in the middle of the bed and put pillows on either side of her, a foot or so away

3. Leave the room and shut the door

4. Go into your bathroom, outside the door, or in the kitchen, and take a few breaths, scream, sob – do whatever you need to do

5. Go back in to your baby when you feel calmer.

Sunbaths

In the first days and weeks, making sunbaths a part of your daily routine is a good way to help your baby move through the normal physiological jaundice that she might have. Vitamin D and ultraviolet rays are helpful for this process.

- You can expose your baby directly to the early morning and late afternoon sun, and to filtered sun through the windows at any time during the day.

- Your baby can be exposed to the sun naked for 10–15 minutes twice a day, but make sure she is warm enough.

- Don't sit in a dark room. Keep your curtains open during the day.

Massage and bath

Newborns crave touch! Babies want massage to be a part of their day. It happens spontaneously during breastfeeding and nappy changing, and while you holding your baby, but it's also nice to incorporate a planned oil massage every day.

Massage has huge benefits for your baby: it

- improves your baby's immune system;

- helps relieve pain of digestion upsets, like colic and gas;

- increases vagal activity, which promotes weight gain;

- stimulates all the developing body systems, including circulatory, digestive, and nervous;

- reduces stress hormones and increases relaxation;

- enhances sensory awareness, supporting more active alert time;

- opens their curled, closed bodies;

- promotes deep sleep; and

- like kangaroo care, it's an awesome support for premature babies.

The benefits for parents include

- enhancing your confidence in handling your baby;
- improving your ability to read your baby's cues;
- giving you a special, focused time with your baby – I usually teach dads!
- providing you with a tool to calm and settle baby; and
- offering a perfect opportunity to introduce your baby's siblings to getting involved in baby's care.

There is a lot of information on the Love Based Birth website, including videos for baby massage.

Do

- Hold him close and swaddle him.
- Wait until the cord falls off (6–10 days after the birth) for the first bath.
- Only use coconut oil on his sensitive skin
- Give him sunbaths twice a day (but only expose him to direct sunlight in the early morning or late afternoon).
- Use cloth diapers at least part time.
- Give him coconut oil massage.
- Use a bucket when bathing him – baby likes to be submerged up to his neck.
- Be kind on yourself. You are not going to get it 'perfect' 100% of the time

- Give him naps on his side – he needs pressure on all sides of his head to avoid his head becoming flat at the back.

- Give him some time on his tummy every day.

- Give his bottom some good air time!

CHAPTER 25

·························

Self-Love And Postnatal Healing

*"Vulnerability is the birthplace of love, belonging, joy, courage,
empathy, and creativity. It is the source of hope,
empathy, accountability, and authenticity.*
Brené Brown, author of *Daring Greatly*

A mum came for biodynamic craniosacral therapy the other day and
sniffed, "Red, there is no epidural for motherhood."

Out of pregnancy, birth and new mothering, many women would
agree that new mothering is the most challenging. Having established
self-love practices and routines during pregnancy, support you during
this period.

In this chapter, we will look at how you can best look after your
healing body and process your experience of birth.

Asking for help

I know you are used to being incredibly self-sufficient and
independent. You have probably lived for 30-something years, are
successful, have had multiple relationships, and traveled the world.
You like to control, you know how you like things, and how to care
for yourself and get what you want. I hear you. Or you might be
younger, in your 20s, and have a good handle on how to look after
yourself and make your way in the world.

It is hard for most women to surrender to asking others for help
during this time. I see it all the time; that is also normal. However, I

encourage you to keep in mind that there is a reason for the saying, 'it takes a village to raise a child.'

Give yourself permission to need help and to ask for support, to ask your partner to make and bring you breakfast, or fill your water bottle, or rub your shoulders, or take baby for a while. Or to call your friend and see if she can pick up a couple things you need from the grocery store.

> "The first few months of motherhood were tough with sleepless nights, but the joy overshadows every struggle. Hang in there. Try and sleep when the baby does. Rest and eat well and be around family and the people you love."
> Nainika, first baby, India

Try using these affirmations or similar ones:

- "I give myself permission to ask for help."
- "I am grateful for the help of others."
- "I accept that I don't need to do everything on my own."

Practicing 'letting go' is essential. Let go of things being a certain way, let go of presenting yourself to the world in a certain way, let go of controlling, let go of the level of efficiency so familiar for you. It is not always easy but an essential practice.

When you start feeling the piles of laundry rising around you, when you haven't yet showered and you wonder if you've even brushed your teeth today, let it go. You haven't failed motherhood, or partnerhood, or selfhood. You are a normal new mum. It will change again. Your old efficiency will come back, possibly even better than ever, because now you have a little one you want to rush back to.

Mothers with toddlers who have their own businesses tell me all the time. "Oh, you just wait; you will get very good at writing a great blog in 15 minutes while the little one is occupied, or keeping your appointments to 30 minutes." The luxury of time and the need for the next level of efficiency automatically changes.

But for now, just breathe, sister. Be here now, and trust it will only be a moment in time.

> "It is a beautifully hectic time! It is a chaotic landing into motherhood. It is an integration phase where all the pieces of you are trying to come back together again, but somehow they just don't fit because you are no longer you anymore. You are a mother now. And there is no going back. Those first few weeks are full with their own emotions, chaos, learnings, lovings, meltdowns, laughter, tears, joy and everything in between. The learning curve is super steep — but it is attainable! So the best thing to do is to really give space for it all. Hibernate, have help, don't make plans and learn how to receive. And make 'patience' be at the top of the list, for everything."
>
> Anonymous, first baby, Singapore

First poo

Most women feel nervous about their first poo after birth. And you'll be happy to know, most women tell me after it happens that it wasn't nearly as bad as they imagined it might be.

Here are a few pointers for supporting healthy elimination after birth:

- Make sure you're drinking enough water – to make up for whatever blood loss you had at the birth.

- Don't eat a lot of constipating foods like white rice, bread and pasta

- Reach for fruits and vegetables.

- Include prunes and dates as a part of your diet.

- When you get the feeling, don't hold it back because of your nerves; the sooner you let it out the better.

  - Relax, use your breath, be gentle, don't force.

  - Avoid using toilet paper on a healing perineum to avoid small particles being caught; use water to clean yourself instead.

- If you are healing from a tear/have stitches, then having a sitz bath once you have finished is a good idea, or rinsing yourself in the shower.

Perineum healing

Whether you have stitches, a tear, or no tear; your perineum will need time to heal. Keep in mind that the vaginal mucosa heals incredibly well, especially with good care.

Here's a list that will help that happen with ease:

- Use natural pads; you will be bleeding for the first several weeks. It will start off like a heavy period for the first few days and then it will start to reduce. You want to get as much airflow as possible, so use a cotton rather than synthetic pad, and one that contains as few chemicals as possible is important. Some of the better brands include Natracare, Natratouch and The Honest Co.

- Light and airflow will help dry up those stitches or heal the nick that wasn't stitched. Spend some time without a pad and panty on; put a towel on your bed and spend an hour or so several times a day (ideally) letting your vagina breathe.

- Calendula is a big orange flower that is well known for its natural antiseptic properties. Using it in tincture form to rinse after you pee will do wonders to support healing and avoid any infection. Just add 10–20 drops to a small mug of warm water and rinse every time you use the toilet.

- Pelvic floor exercise: begin to squeeze your perineum muscles gently as soon as you can find them again; this is beneficial for starting to bring awareness back to your muscles and to increase circulation to the area.

- The less movement in the area the better; going up and down stairs, out for longer walks – all of that will come later but it is not the time for it now. Now is the time for rest, rest, rest, rest.

Sitz baths

Sitz baths are incredibly restorative for your tissues. Gather all the supplies during pregnancy so you can start right away once you are back home, or on day 2 if you are already at home:

1. You need something to soak your bottom in: it can be a specially made plastic insert for the toilet (available in most hospital pharmacies), or a wide, shallow, plastic-rimmed bucket from the market will also work; you could even use the bathtub of an older sibling. You can also sit in your own bathtub, filling it just high enough to come half way up your thighs. (Photos and more information are available on Love Based Birth – search for "sitz bath".)

2. Sitz bath recipe: The following recipe is soothing for you whether you have a tear or not. It supports healing of hemorrhoids and is also a good treatment for persistent candida. Combine

   - Lavender essential oil (or flowers)

   - A handful of Epsom salts

   - Calendula tincture (or flowers)

   - One or two cloves of garlic, peeled and smashed

   - Tea tree oil and grated ginger

If you don't have all those ingredients, use the ones you have. For example, just garlic, lavender and ginger will work well. Depending where you live in the world and what access you have, additional awesome herbs to add include comfrey, rosemary, and uva ursi.

3. Method:

   - Boil a pot of water and turn off the flame.

   - Peel and smash two cloves of garlic

   - Peel and grate a thumb-sized amount of ginger root.

   - Throw in all the non-essential oil/tincture ingredients (garlic/ginger/salt/herbs).

   - Cover and let it steep for 20 minutes

   - Uncover and let cool to a comfortable temperature (or add a little cool water if you want to use it immediately).

   - Pour into your bowl or basin.

   - Add a few drops of essential oils and calendula tincture.

   - Sit with bottom and vagina submerged, and relax for 15–20 minutes.

Do this once or twice a day. You can also use this medicated water in several other ways (minus the garlic):

- Make a squirt bottle and rinse the perineum after peeing

- Make a compress (soak a clean washcloth in the mixture and place on the perineum for 15-20 minutes)

- Some women choose to soak their natural cotton menses pads in the medicated water and then freeze them before using (for women following eastern heating rituals, this will not be appropriate).

Foods that support natural perineum healing include honey and seaweed; these can be placed directly on the perineum.

Hemorrhoids

Unfortunately, hemorrhoids during pregnancy and after are common. Your sitz baths will help to soothe and shrink them. You might also want to try:

- hamamelis homeopathic cream;

- pelvic floor exercises;

- witch-hazel or ginger compress; and

- my favorite home remedy: potatoes. Get a raw potato, peel it, slice it into a wedge or a thick fry, and put it in the freezer for a while. Then get it out and put it against the hemorrhoid. The starch draws out the swelling, and the coolness is very soothing. You can also grate the raw potato and make a small patty to freeze.

Diastasis recti

Your abdominal muscles will take some time to come back together. You can support this by remembering to not overuse or put any strain on them during the fourth trimester. Continue to roll onto your side and push yourself up when getting into and out of bed. You want to use your obliques (the muscles along your sides) first.

Postnatal belly wraps help with this because they restrict your movement. Don't make it so tight that it creates a toothpaste tube effect, putting too much pressure on the pelvic floor.

Processing your birth

Writing can be very helpful after a big experience like birth. Jotting down thoughts, memories and feelings whenever they pop into your mind will help you store the memory outside your head and ensure you don't forget any small details.

Mums tell me all the time how amazed they are at how quickly the details of the birth fade. What remains are the feelings.

Sharing birth stories of birth is very powerful, and you might find it beneficial to tell yours to friends, family or to other mums in postnatal groups. Keep in mind the bubble you had around yourself during pregnancy, though, and remember processing birth with someone pregnant is not a good choice, unless you are telling her positive things, intentionally building her confidence.

I love to share birth stories on Love Based Birth, so you are welcome to send them into me.

Do

- Prepare the supplies you need for postnatal healing in advance.
- Give yourself permission to let the house be messy.
- Let someone look after you and bring you things.
- Stay in bed.
- Ask for what you need.
- Forget about everyone on your phone.
- Accept the support.
- Keep your nails trimmed and take off your nail polish.
- Nap when baby naps.

- Drink plenty of warm fluids.

- Eat foods that are high in iron and protein, and lots of fruit and veg carbs.

- Ask for help – it takes a village to raise a child.

- Stay in your pajamas.

- Take sitz baths.

- Be kind and gentle with yourself, and remember that any new relationship takes work.

CHAPTER 26

Working Through Challenges

"I closed my mouth and spoke to you in a hundred silent ways."
Rumi

Birth and death are the biggest events we can experience in life. For a baby, the two are intertwined. Its birth holds the potential for death, because it is a transition from one reality or one dimension into another; they can't be certain they will make it to the other side, or that there even is another side. Depending how that experience unfolds for baby and what follows immediately after, he might be holding a fight-or flight-response in his little body.

Remember how we talked about sympathetic and parasympathetic automatic nervous systems in the beginning? When the sympathetic is stimulated it produces stress hormones that automatically block the feel-good hormones or oxytocin and endorphins? When birth is filled with many interventions – vacuums or forceps, drugs, separation from mother after the birth, or the life-line (umbilical cord) cut too quickly – there is a greater chance a stress imprint will linger until it gets the chance to be discharged. But it is not just interventionist births that cause babies to hold stress; even the 'gentlest' of births is stressful for baby.

This stress imprint sits on both the emotional and physical planes. Physically, because of the natural compressional forces of birth, and emotionally from the separation of all that is known (the inside of the mother) – feeling the cold, the space, gravity, perhaps with rough or 'routine' handling.

The concept of physical or emotional trauma for the baby after birth is, sadly, still not an accepted norm. Remember we are still just catching up with the idea that babies are even capable of having experiences or feeling pain.

The good news

The good news for babies is that more research and advocacy is coming out all the time, helping us to understand the importance of their experience.

Babies amaze me every day with how quickly they can release compression and stress from their systems. If given an opportunity to work with it early on, when they are still so watery, they can let go of it with simple suggestions – unlike by the time we are adults, our birth stress and life traumas are deeply woven into the fabric of our bones and connective tissues. It will naturally take longer to release.

There are a few things each one of us can do without any specific training.

Validate baby's experience

I attended a birth recently where the baby was gently caught by her father on the bathroom floor of her house. The labor was several hours long, and Mum was relaxed and doing an incredible job working with her oxytocin and breath to bring her out. Baby was gently passed straight from Dad into the waiting arms of her mum where she stayed, and her cord was cut only several hours later. As support people, we stayed on the periphery, available if we were needed.

And boy did that little baby wail – for nearly the entire first hour. She sobbed and shouted uncontrollably. She shook her little fists and shouted her story. She was clearly angry about the whole thing and wanted everyone to know it.

What do you think the mum did? "Shushed" her? Looked around, worried, for someone to tell her what was wrong? Started to panic that her baby didn't like her? No. Her response was one we can all learn from.

She simply heard her daughter, validated her, and reassured her.

"I know it's so bright out here. Are you cold? I know it was such scary, hard work being born. That must have been hard on your perfect beautiful little head. I know, tell me all about it. You are here with me now. I have always loved you. I will always be here for you. It's OK. You are safe." She kissed her over and over, nuzzled her to her breast. Her body was enveloping her energetically, reassuring her that she was very much a connected part of the whole.

Those moments there on the bathroom floor were profound and powerful: a mother's response so compassionate, strong and present; a mother given the space to do for her baby what felt completely natural for her.

As I sat there leaning against the bathroom doorway, holding back my own streaming tears, it all made sense. There was a magic in the room, a sweet, sticky, thick blanket of liquid love filling up each of our nervous systems. I could feel the importance and the healing impact of this moment for that mother and child, and for each one of us in the room.

At the same time, there was grief in my heart for all the babies born all over the world at that same moment who didn't have such strong, confident mothers – babies who were shushed, who felt they didn't have the right to be angry or upset or sad or confused, who understood for the first time that expressing feelings is not something done here in this realm.

Validate baby's experience, while in the womb, and once in your arms; they will love it. "She knows. She hears me! She is here. *I am safe.*"

One of my favorite things about my husband is how good he is at validating my experience, showing me he hears me. He might not understand me, but he sees that whatever it is that is making me cry is real for me. He doesn't even need to say anything, he just pulls me close. Usually, once my sobs stop, he asks if I want to talk about it, and I either do or I don't. Often it is after a birth. Several times it was while writing this book. The opportunities to be embraced and loved are always popping up if we don't suppress them.

Communicating with eye contact

Another way to help babies release stress from their nervous systems is through eye contact. You are probably familiar with the saying, "One look is worth a thousand words". This is even truer for babies because they are primarily connected to their sensing abilities rather than to the rationalizing neocortex that we live in. They are way ahead of us at reading and understanding non-verbal communication.

When your baby looks straight into your eyes, you might feel like you are looking into another universe and surprise yourself at how long you can gaze into those eyes. Try communicating with your eyes that you care. Show compassion with your eyes; tell them you understand, that they are accepted and loved and perfect exactly as they are, that there is plenty of space in the world for them. This empathetic attunement will gently begin to ease their nervous system from that fight-or-flight overdrive into more settled harmony and balance.

> "I'm proud of the fact that I stayed fit and healthy throughout my pregnancy and formed a bond with my baby before he was born. I can see it in his eyes that he knows me. I am also so proud that I gave birth naturally and peacefully without much intervention to give my baby the best start at life."
> Melissa, first baby, South Africa/Singapore

I can give you thousands of examples of this, on buses, planes, trains, on the streets: babies always seem to find my eyes. Those little eyes always want to have reflected the essence of what we all instinctively come in expecting from life: love.

Professional support

In Section 1, I encouraged you to seek out bodywork to ensure your pelvis is aligned and mobile, helping reduce pregnancy discomforts and birth complications. Again, in the postnatal period, I believe it plays an important role for both you and your baby.

Here is a list of scenarios you could face, and if you do, I encourage you to seek out the professional support of someone recommended who does body alignment work as soon as you can. It might be biodynamic craniosacral therapy, or, similar but with more manual manipulation, craniosacral therapy, osteopathy, or chiropractic

- Vacuum or forceps used at birth

- Caesarean birth

- You have pelvic instability or pain in your "tailbone"

- Baby favors one side of his head (for example, he always likes to look to the right)

- Baby is not latching well – you have sore nipples, a fussy baby, slow weight gain, and problems with milk supply

- Baby had a tongue-tie release

- Baby given the label of "colicky" or "high-needs"

- Baby has a "flat head"

- Baby doesn't seem comfortable engaging

- Baby spent time in intensive care

Biodynamic craniosacral therapy

I would love to see every woman and baby on the planet receive a biodynamic craniosacral therapy (BCST) session after birth, regardless of what type of birth they had, and here's why.

BCST is a bodywork that uses light touch to help the nervous system come into a state of balance. It gently straightens out kinks or bends along the physical structure of the body from the membrane system surrounding the brain and spinal cord, to the fascia and bones, and everything in between.

When our bodies are aligned physically, we naturally have access to greater vital force; babies want that, and mums need it. It is such a gentle and beautiful "reset".

Most babies hold tension in their bodies from being in that cramped compartment for a long time, maybe always with the same side of their head squeezed up against the pubic bone. And for mums, BCST supports the body to rest deeply and integrate the new information it has received from the birth process. Often after birth, mums feel like they have been expanded, energetically fragmented. BCST brings a noticeable and often profound renewed sense of peace, connection and "OK-ness" from within for both mum and baby.

"BCST was something I did pre-pregnancy to re-calibrate my body, so naturally, postnatally, I gravitated towards it. As a new mom, after the elation of birth comes the reality of motherhood, which surrounds you with much love and joy, but oh soooo tiring at times. BCST helped my nervous system take a breath and helped my baby ease into the elements of the real world. Even the easiest birth can take its toll on the body and BCST is a very gentle approach to help the body heal."

Anonymous, third baby, Australia/Singapore

Other common reasons mums come to see me after birth for a BCST session, apart from those mentioned above, include baby...

- seeming 'uncomfortable' in her body
- having digestive discomfort
- crying more than expected
- seeming uncomfortable with touch
- seeming anxious, hyper-aroused
- having a strong reaction against tummy time
- having problems breastfeeding
- having troubles sleeping

... and they themselves

- having discomfort – usually in the "tailbone"
- feeling unsettled by the birth (sometimes with nightmares)
- feeling overwhelmed, nervous or anxious
- not feeling a connection to their baby

If you have practitioners in your area, I encourage you to seek out someone who comes highly recommended. You might be surprised how quickly the situation can be resolved.

The following are two potential challenges that can occur in the fourth trimester (or beyond) that deserve a mention:

Trouble coping

If you are feeling more overwhelmed, nervous or anxious than you expected, if you are crying a lot, very angry or generally finding it hard to cope, then know you are not alone. Please reach out for help. Postnatal anxiety or depression is common and no longer a taboo subject. You could check whether your PCP, your doula, or anyone else who was on your support team pre-or postnatally, for resources to help you.

The sooner you seek help, the faster you will get the support you need.

Tongue tie

I recommend finding out a little about this prenatally and then having someone look at your baby's tongue if you are having latching problems. It is becoming more common for lactation support people to know how to check a baby's tongue, but if you don't have anyone in your area, I have included some online resources at the back of the book.

I am seeing more tongue ties affecting breastfeeding in my practice than previously. I have a few theories as to why this is, but I will save that for the second edition of this book!

Some babies need to have their tongue tie clipped, and it is a relatively straightforward process. You will need good follow-up support afterwards to help re-train baby's tongue.

········
Do
········

- Seek out a body worker for your postnatal team.

- Ask for help if you are having troubles coping.

- Remember to think of baby's tongue if your latch is not improving.

Wishing you love, joy and magic as you continue along the road to new motherhood! You are doing a wonderful job turning up and staying open, your baby is very blessed.

Further Resources

Books

Brown, B. (2015). *Daring Greatly: How the courage to be vulnerable transforms the way we live, love, parent, and lead.* London: Penguin Life. (Kindle, audiobook, CD and MP3 versions available)

Dick-Read, G. (2004, sixth edition). *Childbirth Without Fear: The principles and practice of natural childbirth.* London: Pinter & Martin.

Gaskin, I.M. (2008). Ina May's Guide to Childbirth. London: Vermilion.

Goer, H. (1995). *Obstetric Myths versus Research Realities.* Westport, CT: Praeger Publishers. (Kindle edition available)

Gurmukh (2003). *Bountiful, Beautiful, Blissful: Experience the Natural Power of Pregnancy and Birth with Kundalini Yoga and Meditation.* New York: St Martin's Press. (Kindle edition available)

Roar Behind the Silence; why kindness, compassion and respect matter in maternity care Publisher: Pinter & Martin

Odent, M. (2004). *The Caesarean.* London: Free Association Books.

Odent, M. (1999). *The Scientification of Love.* London: Free Association Books.

Renfrew, M., Fisher, C. and Arms, S. (2004). Bestfeeding: How to breastfeed your baby. Berkeley, CA: Celestial Arts.

Sears, W. and Sears, M. (2013, revised edition). *The Baby Book: Everything you need to know about your baby from birth to age two.* New York: Little, Brown and Company. (Audio book and CD and MP3 versions available)

Simkin, P. (2013, 4th edition). *Birth Partner: A complete guide to childbirth for dads, doulas, and all other labor companions.* Boston: Harvard common Press. (Kindle edition available)

Spirit Babies: How to Communicate with the child you are meant to have – Walter Makichen

The Uterine Health Companion: A Holistic Guide to Lifelong Wellness – Eve Agee

Verny, T. and Weintraub, P. (2000). *Nurturing the Unborn Child: A nine-month program for soothing, stimulating and communicating with your baby.* Olmstead Press. (Kindle edition available)

Verny, T. and Weintraub, P. (2003). *Pre-Parenting: Nurturing your child from conception.* New York: Simon & Schuster.

Wirth, F. (2001). *Prenatal Parenting: The complete psychological and spiritual guide to loving your unborn child.* New York: ReganBooks.

Nobody Ever Told Me (or my Mother) That!: Everything from Bottles and Breathing to Healthy Speech Development by Diane Chapman Bahr

Find many more recommended books on LoveBasedBirth.com.

Movies

Microbirth (2014), directed by Toni Harman and Alex Wakeford, UK. http://microbirth.com

In Utero (2015), written and directed by Kathleen Man Gyllenhaal, USA. http://www.inuterofilm.com

Toxic Baby (2016), written and directed by Penelope Jagessar Chaffer, USA.

https://www.youtube.com/watch?v=EjYVr5zbBHc

Online Resources:

Positive Pregnancy and Birth

Love Based Birth : www.loveBasedbirth.com

Birth Without Fear : www.birthwithoutfearblog.com

The Positive Birth Movement: www.positivebirthmovement.org

Orgasmic Birth : www.orgasmicbirth.com

One World Birth : www.oneworldbirth.net

Midwifery Today : www.midwiferytoday.com

Childbirth Connection : www.childbirthconnection.org

Prenatal Parenting:

www.birthPsychology.com

Breastfeeding:

Dr Jack Newman: www.breastfeedinginc.ca

La Lèche League: www.llli.org

Kelly Mom : www.kellymom.com

Breastfeeding Basics : www.breastfeedingbasics.com

Dr Sears: www.askdrsears.com

Tongue Tie

Tongue Tie Institute:

http://www.tonguetieinstitute.com

Tongue Tie: From confusion to clarity

http://tonguetie.net

Craniosacral Therapy

Biodynamic Craniosacral Therapy Association of North America: www.craniosacraltherapy.org

International Institute of Craniosacral Balancing: www.icsb.ch

Skin-to-skin contact studies:

The Touch Institute: http://www6.miami.edu/touch-research/

https://www.ncbi.nlm.nih.gov/pubmed/17542814

https://www.aap.org/en-us/about-the-aap/aap-press-room/Pages/Skin-to-Skin-Contact-with-Baby-in-Neonatal-Unit-Decreases-Maternal-Stress-Levels.aspx?nfstatus=401&nftoken=00000000-0000-0000-0000-000000000000&nfstatusdescription=ERROR%3a+No+local+token

http://www.ncbi.nlm.nih.gov/pubmed/17869557

* * *

If you are birthing in a hospital and inspired to be a part of the global movement of parents and professionals educating and spread awareness of "motherbaby"-friendly practices, including promoting skin-to-skin contact, here are more great resources. Consider meeting with the person in charge of hospital policy.

Improving Birth Coalition: www.motherfriendly.org

Check for The Mother-Friendly Childbirth Initiative (MFCI)

WHO/UNICEF Baby-friendly Hospital Initiative (BFHI): www.who.int/nutrition/topics/bfhi/en/

Acknowledgements

I am deeply grateful to everyone who has supported this project from its conception through to birth.

First and foremost, to my husband and companion in life Ross for his steadfast belief both in me and my work in the world. A belief that is paramount in inspiring me to push the boundaries of comfort to do things like write a book. Thank you for always being such an incredible sounding board and coping with love and presence to the rollercoaster that accompanied this process at times.

To the mothers, with gratitude, who shared their personal experiences with you inside these pages Stacey Lee, Freji, Miranda, Kyra, Dao, Nicky, Yvonne, Lori, Tammy, Nada, Catherine, Nainika, Tanishq, Mary-Signe, Kelly, Aurore, Kasturi, Nicole, Sarah, Bea, Melissa, Andrea, Jasmine, Germaine, Tonia, Teresa, Amanda, Marie, Ikin, Laura, Caroline, Filza and Amber.

To my writing accountability group who kept my fingers tapping during the initial draft stage. To all the early readers who gave me invaluable feedback including my friends, clients and colleagues Amber Sawyer, Sarah Shaw, Arati Davis, Nora Kropp, Priyanka Idicula and Shiela VanDerveer. To the wider world of professionals in the world of birth including Lesley Page, Jan Tritten, Debra Pascali-Bonaro, Dr Paul Tseng, Dr J Ravichandran and Sheena Byron all your encouraging words and feedback keep me going!

Extra special thank you to Amber Sawyer a woman of exceptional intuition and insight who gave hours of time in the first copy edit on a tight timeline. May you be blessed a thousand-fold, dear sister!

To Josh and Daphne for your belief and support to get this to a publisher.

To my awesome publishers at Rethink Press, Lucy McCarraher, Joe Gregory and my editor Verity Ridgman. Your support and patience has been incredible. Lucy, I am so grateful we met, it was your inspiration and push that convinced me this book might actually be possible. I am so grateful for all your guidance along the way.

To my teachers, including all the couples I have worked with over the past twelve years, who have shared their most intimate moments with me and taught me everything I know. To the midwives at the Northern New Mexico Midwifery Centre, Joan, Kristen, Kiersten and Emma, who were there encouraging me in the beginning when I first began this incredible work. To Kavi and Bhadrena Gemin, my Biodynamic Craniosacral teachers and mentors – you opened my eyes and heart to a whole new dimension of what is possible in the body and I thank you.

To my own parents who gave me the incredible gift of life and love.

To the presence of my little one who has been silently encouraging me with nudges and kicks from its private cosmos in my body while I sat for many hours writing. It has been such an honor to share this process with you, my love, I know you have felt every celebration and setback right along with me. Thank you for your sweet presence. And speaking of sitting: to my wonderful body workers who have kept me checking in with my posture and giving me body alignment love as my body expanded along with the pages of this book.

To *you*, reader, for picking up this book and making a commitment to get present with the epic journey from woman to mother, may you be blessed with a deep well of strength and self-love along the way.

Above all to the divine who continues to gently guide and encourage me along this path, giving me the opportunity and energy to share with all of you and birth this book into being.

I am deeply grateful and bow humbly to each one of you.

The Author

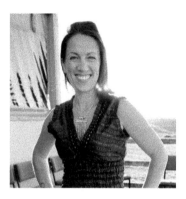

Red Miller is a Birth Consultant, Midwife, Biodynamic Craniosacral therapist, birth geek and the founder of Love Based Birth. She works with women during their journey from pre-conception to new motherhood, helping them to have positive, informed experiences.

Originally from Canada, and trained in the USA, Red has been settled in Asia for ten years offering her expertise throughout Asia and other parts of the world, including Singapore, Malaysia, India, Nepal, Thailand, and Cambodia. Her extensive international experience consulting as a Midwife and supporting local communities has given her a strong understanding of the local as well as global issues facing women and families in birth today in both rural and urban contexts.

She loves working in humble rural rice fields as much as vibrant cities and dreams of every woman having access to information and respectful health care regardless of her background or situation.

In 2010, she co-founded a birth center run by midwives in Kerala, India, called Birthvillage and remains on the board of directors. A pioneer in her field, Red was the consulting, attending midwife for the first water babies in states of Kerala, India and Johor, Malaysia.

Part her big vision is to change the way society views birth. She believes once women start demanding their right to birth their babies in love and respect, and we start to see more babies born that way, a great positive shift will occur in every community and culture.

You can see more of her work here:

www.lovebasedbirth.com

www.pregnancymoon.com

Facebook: Love Based Birth

Lightning Source UK Ltd.
Milton Keynes UK
UKHW02f1147110918
328697UK00003B/22/P